5

NUTRITION AND DIET RESEARCH PROGRESS

FOOD AWAY FROM HOME AND FOOD AT HOME

DEMAND AND NUTRITIONAL QUALITY RESEARCH

NUTRITION AND DIET RESEARCH PROGRESS

Additional books in this series can be found on Nova's website under the Series tab.

Additional E-books in this series can be found on Nova's website under the E-book tab.

NUTRITION AND DIET RESEARCH PROGRESS

FOOD AWAY FROM HOME AND FOOD AT HOME

DEMAND AND NUTRITIONAL QUALITY RESEARCH

SHANE BAUER
EDITOR

New York

For permission to use material from this book please contact us:
Telephone 631-231-7269; Fax 631-231-8175
Web Site: http://www.novapublishers.com

Library of Congress Cataloging-in-Publication Data

ISBN: 978-1-62808-122-0

Published by Nova Science Publishers, Inc. † New York

CONTENTS

PREFACE

Food away from home (FAFH) is a sizable component of total food consumption and the nutritional intake of U.S. adults and children. FAFH also, therefore, constitutes a large and growing portion of the food budget. In 2009, the annual average household expenditure on FAFH was $2,619 or approximately 41 percent of the food budget for an average U.S. household, compared with $1,320, or approximately 29 percent of the food budget in 1984. Recent findings suggest that FAFH may contribute significantly to obesity and poor dietary quality in the United States. Given the potential significance of FAFH for dietary quality and nutrition, policies designed to influence nutritional outcomes should address the role of FAFH. This book estimates the demand for disaggregated FAFH and Food at Home (FAH) products, as elements of an unconditional system of demand equations in a two-stage budgeting process. Statistically significant cross-price relationships, between and within groups of foods, using the first and second stage estimates, underscore the potential usefulness of considering all foods, not just a subset of foods, in evaluating policies targeting nutrition and health outcomes.

Chapter 1 - Food away from home (FAFH) comprises nearly half of all U.S. consumer food expenditures. Hence, policies designed to influence nutritional outcomes would be incomplete if they did not address the role of FAFH. However, because of data limitations, most studies of the response of food demand to policy changes have ignored the role of FAFH, and those studies that have included FAFH have treated it as a single good. We, therefore, estimate demand for 43 disaggregated FAFH and food-at-home (FAH) products, using a 2-stage budgeting framework. We find that the demands for disaggregated FAFH products differ in price responsiveness and tend to be more sensitive to changes in food spending patterns than FAH products. Many foods are found to have statistically significant substitution and complementary relationships within and among food groups. Predicted changes in quantities based on our estimates that include all goods and services and those estimates that include only a subset of foods differ substantially, implying that evaluations of health and nutrition policy based on elasticities of demand for only a subset of goods may be misleading.

Chapter 2 - Food prepared away from home (FAFH)—whether eaten in restaurants, fast-food and other locations, or as take-out or delivery to be eaten at home—is now a routine part of the diets of most Americans, accounting for 41 percent of food expenditures and 32 percent of caloric intake.

This report analyzes data on individuals 2 years of age and older from two national food consumption surveys (one conducted in 1977-78 and another in 2005-08) to assess changes in the consumption and nutritional quality of FAFH versus food prepared at home (FAH). In the past three decades, FAH has changed more in response to dietary guidance, becoming significantly lower in fat content and richer in calcium, whereas FAFH did not. In 2005-08, FAFH was also higher in saturated fat, sodium, and cholesterol and lower in dietary fiber than FAH. The increased popularity and lower nutritional quality of FAFH is prompting new health promotion strategies, such as menu labeling.

In: Food Away from Home and Food at Home
Editor: Shane Bauer
ISBN: 978-1-62808-122-0

Chapter 1

THE DEMAND FOR DISAGGREGATED FOOD - AWAY-FROM-HOME AND FOOD-AT-HOME PRODUCTS IN THE UNITED STATES*

Abigail M. Okrent and Julian M. Alston

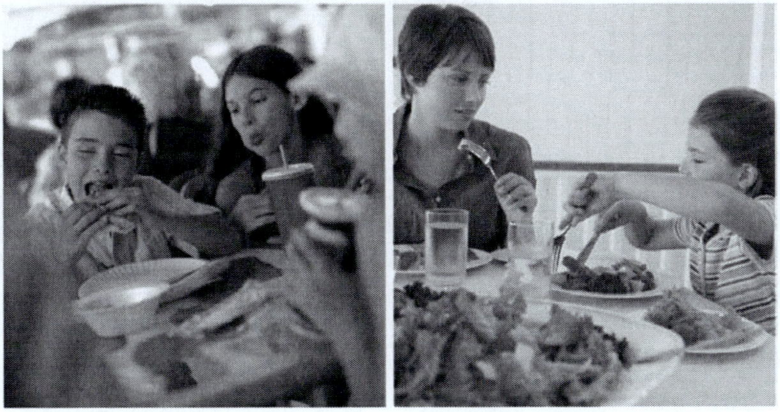

Cover photo credit: Shutterstock.

* This is an edited, reformatted and augmented version of United States Department of Agriculture, Economic Research Service, Economic Research Report Number 139, dated August 2012.

Abstract

Food away from home (FAFH) comprises nearly half of all U.S. consumer food expenditures. Hence, policies designed to influence nutritional outcomes would be incomplete if they did not address the role of FAFH. However, because of data limitations, most studies of the response of food demand to policy changes have ignored the role of FAFH, and those studies that have included FAFH have treated it as a single good. We, therefore, estimate demand for 43 disaggregated FAFH and food-at-home (FAH) products, using a 2-stage budgeting framework. We find that the demands for disaggregated FAFH products differ in price responsiveness and tend to be more sensitive to changes in food spending patterns than FAH products. Many foods are found to have statistically significant substitution and complementary relationships within and among food groups. Predicted changes in quantities based on our estimates that include all goods and services and those estimates that include only a subset of foods differ substantially, implying that evaluations of health and nutrition policy based on elasticities of demand for only a subset of goods may be misleading.

Summary

What Is the Issue?

Food away from home (FAFH, including limited-service and full-service restaurants) constitutes a large and growing portion of the food budget: in 2009, the annual average household expenditure on FAFH was $2,619, or approximately 41 percent of the food budget for an average U.S. household, compared with $1,320, or approximately 29 percent of the food budget in 1984. Because FAFH comprises a sizable share of total food expenditures and nutritional intake for an average American, disregarding the relationships between FAFH and any other subset of foods may produce misleading results for formulating nutrition and health policy. Many studies have excluded or inadequately represented FAFH, such that the estimates only partially capture the effects of policy-induced food price changes on consumer demand and nutrition.

Those analyses that included all goods and services treated FAFH as a composite good, but disaggregated products in FAFH might differ from one another in terms of responsiveness to price- and income-led expenditure changes, nutritional characteristics, or both. Little is known about how demands for different types of FAFH respond to price changes, but a handful of studies have found that demand responds to changes in income differently for full-service food than it does for limited-service food.

What Did the Study Find?

Statistically significant cross-price relationships exist between and within groups of foods. Evidence suggests that demands for FAFH products differ from demands for food-at-home (FAH) products. Further, FAFH products differ among one another in their nutritional characteristics, quality, and responsiveness to changes in prices and expenditure. Specific findings related to cross-price relationships and consumer demand for FAFH include:

- The demands for disaggregated FAFH products tend to be more sensitive to income-induced changes in total expenditures than are FAH products. This finding may explain why the budget share for FAFH products dipped during the recent recession, while the budget shares for many FAH products increased. During December 2007-June 2009, monthly total expenditures fell 0.51 percent for the average American. In addition, the prices of most FAH products, which are mostly gross substitutes for FAFH products, fell relative to the prices of the FAFH products. Hence, income-induced changes in total expenditures and the relative affordability of FAH versus FAFH products caused demand for FAFH to fall.
- The demand for full-service FAFH responds much more readily to price changes than does the demand for limited-service FAFH and other FAFH (including vending machines, mobile food vendors, and school and employee sites).
- Compared with the demands for foods commonly deemed "unhealthy" (e.g., cheese, white bread, cakes and cookies, frozen foods), the demands for many products commonly deemed "healthy" (fruits and vegetables, nonwhite bread, fish, and seafood) tend to be much less responsive to price changes. For example, the demand for nonwhite bread is much less price-elastic than the demand for white bread, and the demand for cookies and cakes is one of the most price-elastic.
- Many of these "healthy" and "unhealthy" foods show statistically significant substitution and complementary relationships within and

among food groups—a finding that complicates any analysis trying to predict the effects of policy-induced price changes on food demands and nutritional outcomes.

- Using forecasts of price and total expenditure changes between 2011 and 2012 to predict food consumption changes over the same span, we found that predictions based on estimates of (conditional) demand elasticities that ignore the total effects of substitutions and complementarities differ substantially—sometimes even taking opposite signs—from predictions based on estimates of (unconditional) demand elasticities that include all goods and services. For example, consumption of each disaggregated dairy product was predicted to *increase* approximately 0.5-1 percent in 2012 when using unconditional demand elasticities, but to *decrease* a similar amount according to conditional elasticities. Similar contradictions in forecast changes in consumption between the two sets of demand elasticities are found for pork, poultry, eggs, sugar and sweets, and frozen foods.
- The substantial cross-price relationships between products in different groups suggest that nutrition policy analysis based on demand elasticities for small groups of products is likely to be misleading.

How Was the Study Conducted?

Using the 1998–2010 Consumer Expenditure Survey diary section, we constructed a monthly time series of household expenditures by aggregating detailed weekly expenditure data into 43 products (i.e., 3 FAFH products, 38 FAH products, alcoholic beverages, and a nonfood composite), and then averaged these data over households for a given month. We then matched the average monthly expenditures to monthly consumer price indices.

We estimated demand for the 43 products using 2-stage budgeting, where the representative consumer allocates expenditures for market goods and services to groups of goods in the first stage, and then chooses products within each group of goods in the second stage. First, we estimated demand for eight food groups (cereals and bakery products, dairy, meat and eggs, fruits and vegetables, nonalcoholic beverages, other FAH, and FAFH/alcoholic beverages), and a nonfood composite good. Second, we modeled the second-stage allocation of expenditures on the eight food groups as weakly separable groups—a structure that allowed us to estimate demand for goods in a given group without considering demand for goods in other groups.

Using demand elasticity estimates from the first- and second-stage allocations, we approximated "unconditional" demand elasticities, which consider the total expenditure for all goods and services. We then computed the changes in food quantities implied by forecasted changes in prices and personal consumption expenditures between 2011 and 2012. The computation used the two sets of demand elasticities and compared the simulated changes to show the influence of intergroup substitution on measures of changes in total nutritional intake.

INTRODUCTION

Food away from home (FAFH) is a sizable component of total food consumption and the nutritional intake of U.S. adults and children. FAFH also, therefore, constitutes a large and growing portion of the food budget: in 2009, the annual average household expenditure on FAFH was $2,619, or approximately 41 percent of the food budget for an average U.S. household, compared with $1,320, or approximately 29 percent of the food budget in 1984 (U.S. Department of Labor, Bureau of Labor Statistics, 2010a).

Recent findings suggest that FAFH may contribute significantly to obesity and poor dietary quality in the United States. Several studies have found that the nutritional content of FAFH is poor compared with food consumed at home (FAH) (Lin, Guthrie, and Frazao, 1999; Jeffrey et al., 2006; Todd, Mancino, and Lin, 2010). In addition, some types of FAFH (e.g., limited-service FAFH, vending machines, and lunch trucks) may be nutritionally worse than others.[1] Consumer proximity to limited-service restaurants—especially proximity to dense concentrations of limited-service restaurants—has been found to contribute to obesity (Chou, Grossman, and Saffer, 2004; Davis and Carpenter, 2009; Currie et al., 2010). Conversely, Binkley (2008) found that—although food from limited-service restaurants tended to be more energy-dense and nutritionally inferior to food from full-service restaurants—meals from limited-service restaurants tended to be smaller. On the whole, the evidence suggests that consuming FAFH may have dramatic effects on dietary quality and body weight and that different types of FAFH may affect dietary quality and individual body weight differently.

Given the potential significance of FAFH for dietary quality and nutrition, policies designed to influence nutritional outcomes should address the role of

FAFH. However, because most studies of the response of food demand to policy changes have disregarded the role of FAFH, the estimates from these studies incompletely reflect changes in food consumption and nutrition resulting from the policy changes. Those studies that included FAFH treated it as a single good, but evidence suggests that FAFH products are heterogeneous in their nutritional characteristics and quality and in how they respond to changes in prices and expenditures.

Some studies have analyzed the relationships between the demands for disaggregated FAFH products and total expenditure or income (i.e., Engel curve analysis), but little is known about the effects of either prices or total expenditure on the demand for disaggregated FAFH products. Only a handful of studies have estimated the effect of price and total expenditure on demand for FAFH as a composite group; to our knowledge, estimates of the effects of prices and total expenditure on demand for disaggregated FAFH have not been published before now. In addition, demand studies that included FAFH as a composite also included fairly aggregated groups of FAH products, whereas some economists have argued that more disaggregated products in terms of "healthy" and "unhealthy" foods would be more useful for policy analysis (Andreyeva, Long, and Brownell, 2009).

In this study, we estimate the demand for disaggregated FAFH and FAH products— including 38 FAH products, 3 FAFH products, alcoholic beverages, and nonfood—as elements of an unconditional system of demand equations in a two-stage budgeting process. We find statistically significant cross-price relationships, between and within groups of foods, using the first- and second-stage estimates—a finding that underscores the potential usefulness of considering all foods, not just a subset of foods, in evaluating policies targeting nutrition and health outcomes. Using estimates of demand elasticities from the first and second stages, we approximate unconditional elasticities of demand. In particular, we find that demand for full-service FAFH differs from its first-stage aggregate: FAFH and alcoholic beverages. Also, demands within the group comprising FAFH and alcoholic beverages differ from each other. Likewise, compared with demand for "healthy" foods, demand for foods commonly deemed "unhealthy" respond differently to own-price changes. Using the unconditional and conditional sets of demand elasticities, we compute predicted changes in consumption of foods implied by forecasts of price changes between 2011 in 2012, compare the results, and discuss the policy implications of basing analysis on estimates derived from conditional versus unconditional demand systems.

PREVIOUS RESEARCH ON MODELING DEMAND FOR FOOD AWAY FROM HOME

In a recent review of the economic literature on the demand for food, Okrent and Alston (2011) found that—in the handful of studies that have estimated the demand for FAFH—FAFH was always treated as a composite food. The earliest studies of food demand that included FAFH as composite good included fairly aggregated foods in other categories as well (Barnes and Gillingham, 1984; Craven and Haidacher, 1987; Nayga and Capps, 1992). Later studies that included disaggregated FAH products and FAFH used fairly restrictive demand systems, which may poorly approximate the actual process that generated the data (Park et al., 1996; Raper et al., 2002).[2]

Piggott (2003); Reed, Levedahl, and Hallahan (2005); and Okrent and Alston (2011) used flexible demand systems with time-series data to estimate demand for FAFH and FAH products in complete demand systems. Piggott (2003) estimated demand for FAH, FAFH, and alcoholic beverages using the nested price independent generalized logarithmic (PIGLOG) demand system and annual data from 1969 to 1999 (i.e., USDA expenditures matched to the Consumer Price Index (CPI)). The nested PIGLOG is very flexible, nesting popular models of demand such as the almost ideal demand system (Deaton and Muellbauer, 1980a) and the indirect translog (Christensen, Jorgenson, and Lau, 1975), as well as globally flexible versions of these models. But again, the estimates of demand elasticities for these three food and beverage groups may be too aggregated to be useful in studies of nutrition policy. Reed, Levedahl, and Hallahan (2005) presented estimates of demand elasticities for an FAFH composite, six FAH products, and a nonfood composite using the semiflexible almost ideal demand system (Moschini, 1998) and the Consumer Expenditure Survey (CEX) aggregated into a quarterly time series matched to the CPI. However, the demands for all of the goods were found to have quite large income elasticities (all in the elastic range), which violates Engel's law. Okrent and Alston (2011) argued that—because unit roots were detected in the logarithmic transformations of the price indexes and budget shares used in their analysis—a differential-demand systems model would be appropriate for modeling demand using those data. They modeled demand for FAFH, alcoholic beverages, eight FAH products, and a nonfood composite using Barten's synthetic model (Barten, 1993; Brown, Lee, and Seale, 1994), which nests four differential-demand systems (i.e., the Rotterdam, National Bureau of Research (NBR), Central Bureau of Statistics (CBS), and differenced linear almost ideal demand system). All of these studies treat FAFH as a single composite good, although the effects of prices and expenditure may differ among individual FAFH products. A few studies analyzed the relationship between demand for disaggregated FAFH products and income or total expenditure, assuming that the price of food from limited-service restaurants relative to food from full-service restaurants would be the same across households. Using different data sets, Byrne, Capps, and Saha (1998) and Stewart et al. (2004) found that income, household size, and labor force participation were statistically significant determinants of expenditure on FAFH for various establishment types. However, to our knowledge, no study before this one has evaluated the effects of changes in prices and total expenditure on demands for disaggregated FAFH products.

Data

Like Reed, Levedahl, and Hallahan (2005) and Okrent and Alston (2011), we use the Consumer Expenditure Survey (CEX) paired with CPIs to estimate the demands for disaggregated FAFH and FAH products, alcoholic beverages, and nonfood. The CEX is a nationwide household survey administered every year since 1984 and designed to represent the total U.S. civilian noninstitutionalized population. The CEX consists of two surveys: a diary survey and a quarterly interview survey. The diary survey collects detailed data on expenditures for frequently purchased items, such as food and apparel, while the interview survey obtains detailed data on expenditures for infrequently purchased items, such as property, automobiles, and major appliances, and on recurring expenses, such as rent, utilities, and insurance premiums. The diary survey collects detailed data on FAH and FAFH expenditures for a 2-week period. The interview survey contains data on expenditures on aggregate food categories, such as FAH and FAFH (U.S. Department of Labor, Bureau of Labor Statistics, 2010b). The CEX diary data are from cross-sections of households and can be aggregated to construct a weekly, monthly, quarterly, or annual time series of average expenditures per consuming unit. Because the CPIs are available monthly and annually, we aggregated the CEX diary data to create a monthly series. When consuming units reported expenditures for a week that straddled 2 months, those expenditures were assigned to the month that included 4 or more of the days in question. Households that did not report purchasing a particular food were assigned a zero. To extrapolate the sample observations to the population, we applied the sample weights calculated by the Bureau of Labor Statistics (BLS). The CEX public microdata are available from 1980 through 2010, but we used a subset of the data since it was only in 1998 that the CEX began publishing detailed data on FAFH (specifically, food from limited-service restaurants, full-service restaurants, vending machines and lunch trucks, employee and school sites, and catered affairs).[3]

We constructed the budget shares as expenditure for each food group divided by total expenditures on all goods and services for the first stage, and as expenditure for each disaggregated food product divided by expenditures for its group for the second stage (table 1). On average, for 1998-2010, nonfood constituted the largest share of the budget for all goods and services at 81 percent, followed by FAFH and alcoholic beverages (8 percent), meat and eggs (3 percent), and other FAH (3 percent). Within the FAFH and alcohol category, food from limited-service and full-service restaurants constituted about 41 percent and 37 percent, respectively, although the average monthly share of limited-service FAFH, within FAFH and alcohol, declined over the entire period (a linear trend of -0.09 percent per month), while the share of full-service FAFH increased (a linear trend of 0.14 percent per month). Other FAFH—which includes food from vending machines and mobile vendors, as well as employee and school sites—constitutes about 7 percent of the expenditure on FAFH and alcohol, and this share has declined by 0.24 percent per month, on average. Expenditure on all of the disaggregated FAFH and alcohol products declined relative to expenditure on total goods and services during the most recent recession (December 2007-June 2009). This finding contrasts starkly with the data on most FAH products, for which expenditure increased as a share of total goods and services during the recession, with the exception of some fruits and vegetables (i.e., bananas, other fresh fruit, and tomatoes), some cereals and bakery products (i.e., white bread, cakes and cookies, and other bakery products), and milk. The budget shares for all foods exhibit considerable month-to-month variation. Expenditure on limited-service FAFH decreased from about 4 percent to 3 percent of the total budget for all goods and services of an average household between 1998 and 2010 (fig. 1). Conversely, the share of the total expenditures for goods and services spent on full-service FAFH grew between 1998 and 2007, but fell thereafter. Expenditures on the FAH products with the largest budget shares likewise seemed to reflect the recession's influence, declining as a share of the total budget on goods and services until 2006, and then increasing thereafter (fig. 2).

Table 1. Summary statistics and trends for budget shares and prices

	Budget shares (%)				Consumer price indexes (Jan. 1999=100)			
			Avg. monthly growth (%)[b]				Avg. monthly real growth (%)[c]	
	Mean[a]	Std. dev.	Jan. 98 -Dec. 10	Dec. 07 - June 09	Mean[a]	Std.dev .	Jan. 98 - Dec. 10	Dec. 07 - June 09
Cereals/bakery	1.66	0.21	-0.12	0.51	114.71	12.90	0.23	0.02
Flour, flour mixes	4.40	0.77	-0.23	1.56	113.84	15.68	0.27	0.05
Breakfast cereals	19.01	1.51	-0.20	0.43	105.40	4.05	0.07	-0.14
Rice, pasta	10.18	1.24	-0.09	1.30	115.89	18.92	0.30	0.09
Non-white bread	11.26	1.01	0.04	0.20	123.93	20.96	0.35	0.14
White bread	7.69	0.73	-0.23	-0.38	122.75	19.73	0.33	0.12
Biscuits, rolls, muffins	9.15	0.87	-0.02	0.52	120.15	17.28	0.30	0.09
Cakes, cookies	17.91	1.62	-0.17	-0.18	113.74	12.60	0.23	0.02
Other bakery products	20.41	1.86	-0.04	-0.02	114.29	10.91	0.20	-0.01
Dairy	1.21	0.11	-0.01	0.03	110.68	11.02	0.28	0.07
Cheese	31.66	2.20	0.07	0.20	111.71	11.53	0.38	0.16
Frozen dairy desserts	17.35	3.00	-0.17	0.32	107.68	7.55	0.18	-0.04
Milk	36.74	2.32	-0.08	-0.94	110.70	13.04	0.22	0.00
Other dairy	14.25	2.15	0.24	0.21	112.11	11.09	0.21	-0.01
Meat and eggs	2.88	0.38	-0.16	0.41	126.17	16.18	0.21	-0.01
Beef	29.09	2.37	-0.22	0.00	135.30	22.95	0.33	0.12
Pork	20.23	1.53	-0.21	0.44	119.61	9.97	0.21	-0.01
Other red meat	13.03	1.19	-0.09	0.00	116.34	11.56	0.21	0.00
Poultry	18.11	1.62	-0.17	0.21	112.85	10.78	0.14	-0.07
Fish	14.75	1.50	-0.07	0.35	111.67	11.51	0.22	0.01

	Budget shares (%)				Consumer price indexes (Jan. 1999=100)			
			Avg. monthly growth (%)[b]				Avg. monthly real growth (%)[c]	
	Mean[a]	Std. dev.	Jan. 98 -Dec. 10	Dec. 07 - June 09	Mean[a]	Std.dev.	Jan. 98 - Dec. 10	Dec. 07 - June 09
Eggs	4.80	0.77	0.06	0.07	116.70	22.64	0.21	0.00
Fruits and vegetables	1.69	0.19	0.06	0.40	113.57	13.54	0.26	0.04
Apples	6.99	1.14	0.01	-0.29	131.99	22.25	0.33	0.12
Bananas	6.57	0.86	-0.11	0.52	110.56	10.99	0.17	-0.04
Citrus	7.84	1.27	0.13	0.34	128.36	25.40	0.36	0.15
Other fresh fruit	17.59	4.90	0.21	-0.29	95.53	11.49	0.18	-0.04
Potatoes	6.64	0.78	0.00	0.61	134.29	26.39	0.40	0.19
Lettuce	4.88	0.39	0.07	0.30	122.06	16.24	0.21	0.00
Tomatoes	6.95	0.75	0.05	-0.37	93.78	15.53	0.27	0.06
Other fresh vegetables	19.43	1.28	0.08	0.14	118.92	15.52	0.28	0.06
Proc. fruits, vegetables	23.10	2.93	0.06	0.69	115.85	14.63	0.26	0.05
Nonalcoholic beverages	0.75	0.09	-0.10	0.53	109.10	7.63	0.14	-0.07
Coffee, tea	17.44	2.42	-0.19	0.18	104.68	10.56	0.19	-0.02
Carbonated beverages	35.07	3.85	-0.88	0.11	113.09	10.40	0.27	0.06
Noncarbonated beverages	45.20	3.66	0.15	-0.63	106.09	5.53	0.11	-0.11
Frozen beverages	2.29	1.10	0.20	0.53	115.02	15.95	0.16	-0.06
Other FAH	2.76	0.34	0.14	0.53	109.81	8.57	0.16	-0.05
Sugar, sweets	18.75	3.28	-0.05	0.44	111.27	10.79	0.20	-0.01
Fats, oils	16.81	1.86	-0.03	0.53	111.73	12.90	0.23	0.02
Soups	5.93	1.16	0.02	0.72	110.46	6.99	0.13	-0.09
Frozen meals	17.15	1.80	0.26	0.23	104.86	4.74	0.09	-0.12
Snacks	3.73	0.39	0.11	0.44	113.16	11.63	0.21	0.00

Table 1. (Continued)

		Budget shares (%)			Consumer price indexes (Jan. 1999=100)			
			Avg. monthly growth (%)[b]				Avg. monthly real growth (%)[c]	
	Mean[a]	Std. dev.	Jan. 98 -Dec. 10	Dec. 07 - June 09	Mean[a]	Std.dev.	Jan. 98 - Dec. 10	Dec. 07 - June 09
Condiments, sauces, season.	15.26	1.14	0.15	0.69	108.56	7.76	0.15	-0.07
Miscellaneous FAH	22.37	3.54	0.41	0.16	107.74	5.84	0.11	-0.10
FAFH and alcohol	8.38	0.75	0.00	0.00	116.41	12.92	0.24	0.03
Alcohol	15.55	2.06	0.05	-0.05	110.90	11.44	0.22	0.01
Full service	37.34	2.71	0.14	-0.22	116.29	12.68	0.24	0.02
Limited FAFH	40.61	3.13	-0.09	-0.24	115.55	11.51	0.25	0.04
Other FAFH	6.51	1.67	-0.24	-0.23	109.71	10.29	0.17	-0.05
Nonfood	80.67	1.58	0.00	-0.06	116.43	11.14	0.21	0.00

Sources: U.S. Department of Labor, BLS, Consumer Expenditure Survey (2010a/b). Notes: Foods in the first stage are highlighted.

FAFH = Food away from home, including limited-service and full-service restaurants.

FAH = Food-at-home.

[a] The mean expenditure shares for the disaggregated products are conditional on the group expenditure.

[b] The average monthly growth rate in the expenditures for the food as a share of total expenditures on goods and services (price) is the coefficient on a linear trend in the ordinary least squares (OLS) regression of the logarithmic transformation of the budget share (price) on the linear trend and a constant.

[c] The real price is the price index for a particular food divided by the consumer price index for all items.

In contrast, the share of total expenditure on other FAH—which consists of sugar and sweets; fats and oils; soups; frozen foods; and condiments, sauces, and gravies—was unaffected by the recession, remaining flat until 2004 and then growing, unabated.

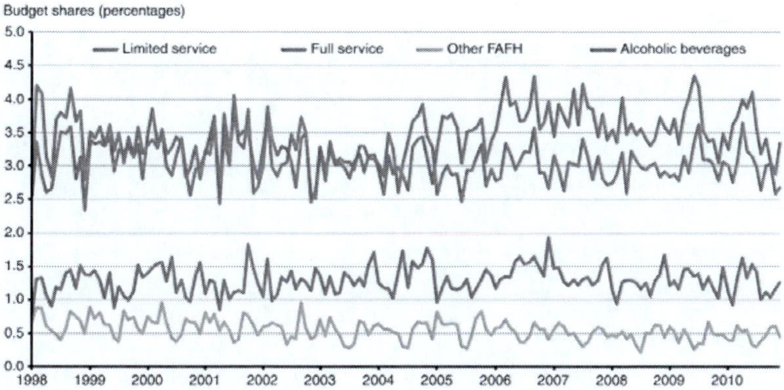

Note: FAFH = Food away from home, including limited-service and full-service restaurants.

Source: Authors' calculations using the Consumer Expenditure Survey (Department of Labor, Bureau of Labor Statistics, 2010a) and the Consumer Price Indexes (Department of Labor, Bureau of Labor Statistics, 2010c).

Figure 1. Monthly household budget expenditures for FAFH and alcohol products as a share of total expenditures on goods and services, 1998-2010.

Most of the food groups in our analysis correspond directly to one of the CPIs. However, two of the food groups—other FAFH and FAFH/alcoholic beverages—correspond to more than one CPI (U.S. Department of Labor, Bureau of Labor Statistics, 2010c). We constructed a composite price index for each of these food groups as a harmonic mean of disaggregated price indexes, each weighted by its first- or second-stage expenditure share. All price indexes are scaled to be equal to 100 in January 1999.

The price indexes for limited-service and full-service FAFH deflated by the CPI for all items seem to track each other, although the commodity price shocks in 2007 and 2008 had a much bigger impact on limited-service FAFH than on full-service FAFH (fig. 3). The growth in both of these real price series is fairly flat until 2008. On the other hand, the real price of other FAFH generally declined until 2008. Of the four products, the real price for alcoholic beverages exhibits the most price variation from month to month, but does not seem to trend up or down over the sample period. Compared to the deflated prices of FAFH, the deflated FAH prices decreased dramatically after the commodity price shocks in 2008 (fig. 4).

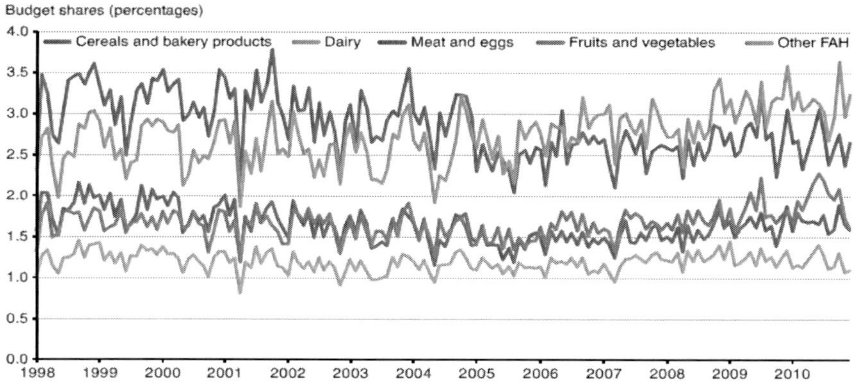

Note: FAH = Food at home

Source: Authors' calculations using the Consumer Expenditure Survey (U.S. Department of Labor, BLS, 2010a) and the Consumer Price Indexes (U.S. Department of Labor, BLS, 2010c).

Figure 2. Monthly household budget expenditures for selected FAH products as a share of total expenditures on goods and services, 1998-2010.

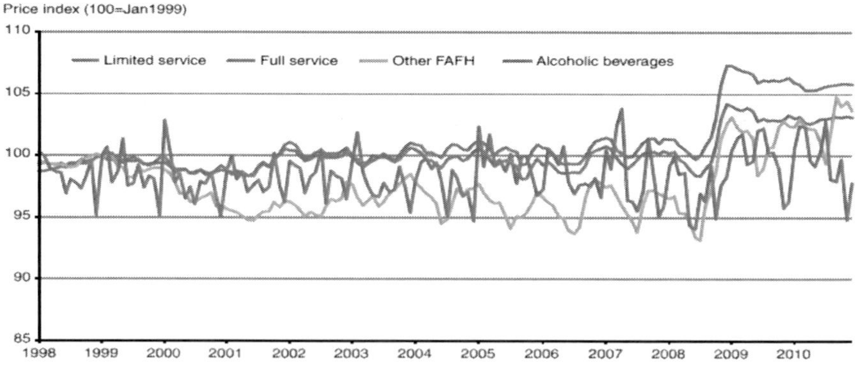

Note: FAFH = Food away from home, including limited-service and full-service restaurants.

Source: Authors' calculations using the Consumer Expenditure Survey (U.S. Department of Labor, BLS, 2010a) and the Consumer Price Indexes (U.S. Department of Labor, BLS, 2010c).

Figure 3. Real prices for disaggregated FAFH and alcohol products, 1998-2010 Price index (100=Jan1999).

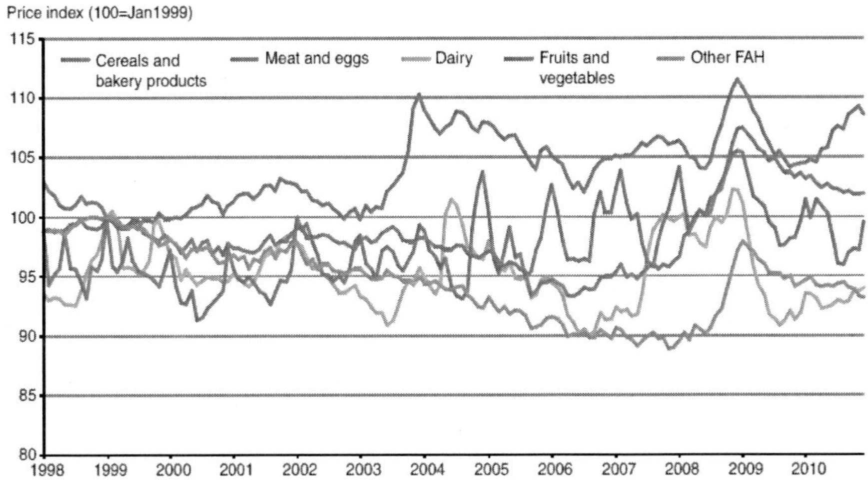

Note: FAH = Food at home.

Source: Authors' calculations using the Consumer Expenditure Survey (U.S. Department of Labor, BLS, 2010a) and the Consumer Price Indexes (U.S. Department of Labor, BLS, 2010c).

Figure 4. Real prices for selected FAH products, 1998-2010 Price index (100=Jan1999).

ESTIMATION APPROACH

Given that we have a limited number of observations and a large number of parameters to estimate, we assume that a representative household purchases goods in a two-stage budgeting process (Strotz 1957, 1959; Gorman, 1959; Barten, 1977), as follows.

First, consumers allocate their budget for all goods and services among composite groups, including six FAH groups, FAFH and alcoholic beverages, and nonfood (fig. 5). Second, assuming that the seven food groups are weakly separable, consumers then choose disaggregated food products within each of the groups, conditional on expenditure for that group. We estimate the first- and second-stage demands for nonfood and disaggregated food products. We then use the first- and second-stage estimates to approximate "unconditional" elasticities of demand for disaggregated food products.[4]

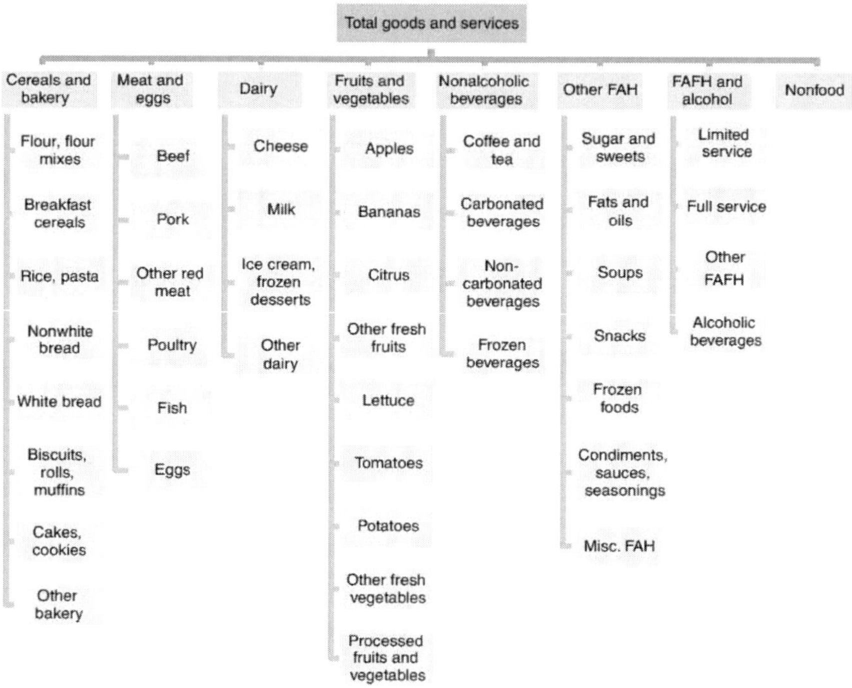

Notes: FAFH = Food away from home, including limited-service and full-service restaurants FAH = Food-at-home.

Demand for market goods and services assumed to be separable from demand decisions about leisure and savings.

Figure 5. Food products within the two-stage budgeting framework.

Estimation of First- and Second-Stage Demand

Since unit roots are often detected in time-series data, Gao and Shonkwiler (1993) suggested working with difference models rather than level-data models because the consequences of differencing when it is not needed are much less serious than those of failing to difference when it is appropriate. Hence, we opted to use the Generalized Ordinary Differential Demand System (GODDS) (Barten, 1993; Eales, Durham, and Wessells, 1997) to estimate demands in both the first and second stages.

The GODDS nests several commonly used differential demand systems, including the Rotterdam model (Theil, 1965; Barten, 1966); the Central

Bureau of Statistics (CBS) model (Keller and van Driel, 1985); the differenced linear almost ideal demand system (DLAIDS) (Deaton and Muellbauer, 1980a); and the National Bureau of Research (NBR) model (Neves, 1987). The GODDS is

$$d\mathbf{w}_n = (c_n + \varphi_1 \mathbf{w}_n) d \ln \mathbf{Q} + \sum_{k=1}^{N} [d_{nk} + \varphi_2 \mathbf{w}_n (\delta_{nk} - \mathbf{w}_k)] d \ln \mathbf{p}_k \tag{1}$$

where c_n and d_{nk} are expenditure and price coefficients to be estimated, respectively; (φ_1 and (φ_2 are nesting coefficients; δ_{nk} is the Kronecker delta; $\mathbf{w}_n$ is a $t \times 1$ vector of expenditure shares for good n; $\mathbf{p}_k$ is a $t \times 1$ vector of prices of good k; and $\mathbf{Q}$ is a $t \times 1$ vector of Divisia volume indexes (see appendix for more details on this model). The values of (φ_1 and φ_2 that generate the various nested models in GODDS are

$\varphi_1 = -1, \varphi_2 = 1$ Rotterdam model (2)
$\varphi_1 = 0, \varphi_2 = 0$ DLAIDS (3)
$\varphi_1 = 0, \varphi_2 = 1$ CBS model (4)
$\varphi_1 = -1, \varphi_2 = 0$ NBR model. (5)

Restrictions from demand theory can also be imposed a priori or tested,

$$\sum_{n=1}^{N} d_{in} = 0, \tag{6}$$

$$\sum_{n=1}^{N} d_{ni} = 0, \sum_{n=1}^{N} c_n = -\varphi_1, \tag{7}$$

$$d_{ik} = d_{ki}, \tag{8}$$

(i.e., homogeneity, adding-up, and symmetry, respectively). The formulas for the price and expenditure elasticities of demand for the GODDS are

$$\eta_{ik} = \frac{d_{ik} - c_i w_k}{w_i} + (\varphi_2 - 1)\delta_{ik} - (\varphi_1 + \varphi_2) w_k, \tag{9}$$

$$\eta_{iM} = \frac{c_i - \varphi_I w_i + w_i}{w_i}. \tag{10}$$

Approximating Unconditional Elasticities of Demand

Many studies model only the second stage of the two-stage budgeting process, and some have argued that the resulting conditional elasticities of demand are a useful approximation to the unconditional elasticities (Capps and Havlicek, 1984; Heien and Pompelli, 1988; Gao and Spreen, 1994). However, the conditions that allow conditional elasticities of demand to approximate unconditional elasticities do not hold empirically.[5] Hence, we approximate the unconditional elasticities of demand by assuming consumers purchase goods in a two-stage budgeting process, and use the first- and second-stage elasticities of demand to approximate the unconditional elasticities of demand.

Carpentier and Guyomard (2001) approximated unconditional elasticities of demand using an approximation to the Slutsky substitution terms that are assumed to be weakly separable. Denoting the superscript as representing the composite group and the subscript as representing the elementary good, they approximated the unconditional Marshallian expenditure (η_{iM}) and price (η_{ij}) elasticities of demand as

$$\eta_{iM} \approx \eta^{I}_{iM}\, \eta^{IM}, \tag{11}$$

$$\eta_{ij} \approx \delta^{IJ} \eta^{I}_{ij} + w^{J}_{j}\, \eta^{I}_{iM}\, \eta^{J}_{jM} (\delta^{IJ} / \eta^{J}_{jM} + \eta^{IJ}) + w^{J}_{j}\, w^{J}\, \eta^{IM}\, \eta^{I}_{iM} (\eta^{J}_{jM} - 1), \tag{12}$$

η^{I}_{iM} = expenditure elasticity for good $i \in I$ conditional on expenditure for group I,

η^{IM} = expenditure elasticity for composite group I with respect to total expenditure, M,

η^{I}_{ij} = Marshallian elasticity of demand for good $i \in I$ with respect to price $j \in J$ conditional on $I = J$,

η^{IJ} = Marshallian elasticity of demand for composite group I with respect to composite price J,

w_j^{rJ} = budget share for good j≍ J conditional on J,

w^{rJ} = budget share for composite group *J*,

$$\delta^{IJ} = \begin{cases} 1, \text{ if } I = J \\ 0, \text{ otherwise} \end{cases}$$

We use the formulas in (11) and (12) and our first- and second-stage estimates of elasticities of demand to approximate unconditional elasticities of demand for disaggregated food products. The approximate unconditional elasticities of demand satisfy the restrictions implied by homogeneity, symmetry, and Cournot and Engel aggregation.

New Estimates of Demand for Disaggregated Food-Away-From-Home and Food-at-Home Products

To estimate the GODDS, we augmented equation (1) in two ways. First, because our data are discrete, we approximated the infinitesimal changes with their discrete counterparts:

$$dw_n \approx \Delta w_n = w_{n,t} - w_{n,t-12}, \forall n = 1,...,N, \tag{13}$$

$$dp_n \approx \Delta \ln p_n = \ln p_{n,t} - \ln p_{n,t-12}, \forall n = 1,...,N, \tag{14}$$

$$d \ln Q \approx \Delta \ln M - \sum\nolimits_{n=1}^{N} \Delta \ln p_n, \text{ where} = (w_{n,t} + w_{n,t-12}), \forall n = 1,...,N. \tag{15}$$

Seale, Marchant, and Basso (2003) recommended twelfth-differencing rather than first-differencing the data when monthly data are used in estimation. In addition, we detected unit roots at seasonal frequencies for many of the logarithmic transformations of the prices and expenditure shares (see appendix tables A.1. and A.2).[6] Second, we included a constant in each equation that acts as a linear trend term when modeling differenced data. To avoid singularity of the variance-covariance matrix, we left out the nonfood equation for the first-stage estimation, and used Engel and Cournot aggregation conditions (i.e., equation (7)) to recover the parameter estimates of nonfood demand; likewise, we left out equations for other bakery products, other dairy, eggs, processed fruits and vegetables, frozen beverages, and miscellaneous FAH in the estimation of the respective second-stage allocations. The GODDS was estimated for the first- and second-stage allocations using iterated feasible generalized least squares, which yield maximum-likelihood estimates of the demand parameters and imply that the system estimates are invariant to which of the equations is deleted (Kmenta and Gilbert, 1968; Barten, 1969).[7]

We first tested whether the data support restrictions associated with any of the nested models (i.e., equations (2)-(5)) using the likelihood ratio statistic. The restrictions associated with the DLAIDS model cannot be rejected for most of the estimated models of second-stage allocations; the model for fruits and vegetables is an exception (table 2). This model implies that the Engel curves of products within these second-stage allocations are of the form used by Working (1943) and Leser (1963) (i.e., $w_n = a_n + \beta_n \ln M$, where M is total expenditure and w_n is the budget share for product n), and both the Slutsky substitution and marginal budget terms vary over time. All of the nesting restrictions on parameters are rejected in the second-stage model of demand for fruits and vegetables, while none of the nesting parameter restrictions is rejected in the second-stage model of demand for dairy.

In the first-stage allocations, the restrictions associated with the NBR and Rotterdam models cannot be rejected; the NBR and Rotterdam models assume constant marginal budget shares. The model restrictions associated with the CBS model, which has price coefficients similar to the Rotterdam model (i.e., constant Slutsky substitution terms) and an income coefficient similar to the DLAIDS, cannot be rejected for the second-stage models of demand for meat and eggs, dairy, and FAFH/alcohol. Hence, because the restrictions associated with multiple nested models cannot be rejected in some cases (as with the estimates of first-stage allocations and second-stage models of demand for dairy and meat/eggs), but are completely rejected in others (as with second-stage model of demand for fruits and vegetables), we present elasticities of demand for the GODDS model for all of the first- and second-stage allocations, including those cases where a more restrictive model could have been used. It has been argued that the GODDS and its reparameterization, Barten's synthetic model, are not merely artificial composites of known differential demand systems, but can be viewed as demand systems in their own right (Eales, Durham, and Wessells, 1997; Matsuda, 2005).

Table 2. Likelihood ratio statistics for nested models

Model	Expenditure group	Likelihood ratio statistic	
Rotterdam (φ1 = -1, φ2 = 1)	Total goods and services	3.37	[0.19]
	Cereals and bakery	19.65	[0.00]
	Meat and eggs	6.57	[0.04]
	Dairy	3.86	[0.14]
	Fruits and vegetables	56.69	[0.00]
	Nonalcoholic beverages	13.38	[0.00]
	Other FAH	17.24	[0.00]
	FAFH and alcohol	12.56	[0.00]
DLAIDS (Differenced linear almost ideal demand system) (φ1 = φ2 = 0)	Total goods and services	15.16	[0.00]
	Cereals and bakery	5.74	[0.06]
	Meat and eggs	0.47	[0.79]
	Dairy	0.83	[0.66]
	Fruits and vegetables	11.55	[0.00]
	Nonalcoholic beverages	3.92	[0.14]
	Other FAH	4.10	[0.13]
	FAFH and alcohol	5.62	[0.06]
CBS (Central Bureau of Statistics) (φ1 = 0, φ2 = 1)	Total goods and services	17.59	[0.00]
	Cereals and bakery	7.14	[0.03]
	Meat and eggs	2.66	[0.26]
	Dairy	2.62	[0.27]
	Fruits and vegetables	14.65	[0.00]
	Nonalcoholic beverages	6.56	[0.04]
	Other FAH	6.17	[0.05]
	FAFH and alcohol	3.81	[0.15]
NBR (National Bureau of Research) (φ1 = -1, φ2 = 0)	Total goods and services	0.50	[0.78]
	Cereals and bakery	18.25	[0.00]
	Meat and eggs	5.33	[0.07]
	Dairy	1.79	[0.41]
	Fruits and vegetables	52.70	[0.00]
	Nonalcoholic beverages	11.26	[0.00]
	Other FAH	15.30	[0.00]
	FAFH and alcohol	14.10	[0.00]

Source: Authors' calculations.

Notes: The bracketed terms are p-values for the null hypothesis that the nesting restrictions are supported by the data.

FAFH = Food away from home, including limited-service and full-service restaurants.

FAH = Food-at-home.

We then tested whether the data supported the restrictions of homogeneity (equation 6) and symmetry (equation 8) from demand theory for the first- and second-stage estimates based on the GODDS (table 3). For the first-stage estimates, homogeneity and symmetry were rejected. Many of the second-stage estimates supported symmetry, except fruits and vegetables and other FAH. Homogeneity is supported only in the nonalcoholic beverage and FAFH/alcoholic beverages second stages.[8] Since we find some support for both symmetry and homogeneity restrictions, we model the first and second stages using the GODDS and with these restrictions.

Last, we tested for first-order autocorrelation in the first- and second-stage estimates (with homogeneity and symmetry restrictions) using the Rao-Breusch-Godfrey test for first-order autocorrelation for the system of equations (Edgarton and Shukur, 1999).[9] We detected first-order autocorrelation in the second-stage estimates for nonalcoholic beverages only. Following Berndt and Savin (1975), we constrained the first-order autocorrelation coefficient to be the same across all equations to preserve adding-up.

We then re-estimated the nonalcoholic beverages' second stage with a correction for first-order autocorrelation, using iterated feasible generalized nonlinear least squares.[10]

First-Stage Estimates of Demand Elasticities for Composite Goods

The GODDS model seems to fit the monthly data well. The single-equation R2 statistics ranged between 0.58 for FAFH and alcohol and 0.77 for cereals and bakery products (table 4). The system R^2 based on Bewley, Young, and Colman (1987) is 0.17, indicating that about 17 percent of the variation in the dependent variables in the first stage can be explained by the price terms in the GODDS model.[11] The constant is significant in the equations for cereal and bakery products, meat and eggs, and fruits and vegetables; in particular, the estimated constants indicate trends of increasing consumption for cereals and bakery products and meat and eggs, and decreasing consumption for fruits and vegetables.

All of the own-price elasticities for the first-stage allocations are negative, which is consistent with demand theory. Most of the own-price elasticities of demand are significant at 10 percent except for dairy, for which the estimate is very small, indicating a very inelastic demand.

Table 3. Goodness of fit, tests of autocorrelation, and restrictions from demand theory for all first- and second-stage estimates based on GODDS (Generalized Ordinary Differential Demand System)

Conditional on expenditure for	System R_2	Rao- Breusch-Godfrey statistic	Likelihood ratio statistics for restrictions from demand theory					
			Symmetry		Homogeneity		Symmetry and homogeneity	
Total goods and services	0.15	0.64	49.22	[0.00]	22.44	[0.00]	61.28	[0.00]
Cereals and bakery	0.07	0.65	23.78	[0.31]	23.64	[0.00]	45.16	[0.02]
Meat and eggs	0.18	0.30	23.28	[0.05]	18.06	[0.00]	39.78	[0.00]
Dairy	0.20	1.47	4.96	[0.17]	11.92	[0.00]	13.24	[0.05]
Fruits and vegetables	0.08	0.93	60.32	[0.00]	17.02	[0.03]	77.84	[0.00]
Nonalcoholic beverages	0.09	2.19	5.04	[0.17]	0.20	[0.98]	10.50	[0.11]
Other food at home	0.07	0.57	53.00	[0.00]	21.26	[0.00]	74.66	[0.00]
Food away from home/alcohol	0.09	1.85	3.26	[0.35]	4.14	[0.25]	6.28	[0.39]

Source: Authors' calculations.

Notes: The bracketed terms are p-values for the likelihood ratio tests of the null hypothesis that the restrictions from demand theory are supported by the data. The Rao-Breusch-Godfrey statistic is approximately distributed $F(p,q)$, of which the 5% critical value is (i) 1.39 for the first-stage model, with $p = 49$ and $q = 609$, and, in the second-stage allocations (ii) 1.39 for cereals and bakery, with $p = 49$ and $q = 609$; (iii) 1.46 for meat and eggs, with $p = 25$ and $q = 466$; (iv) 1.88 for dairy, with $p = 9$ and $q = 290$; (v) 1.31 for fruits and vegetables, $p = 64$ and $q = 676$; (vi) 1.88 for nonalcoholic beverages, with $p = 9$ and $q = 319$; (vii) 1.67 for other FAH, with $p = 16$ and $q = 536$; and (viii) 1.88 for FAFH and alcoholic beverages, with $p = 9$ and $q = 288$.

Table 4. First-stage uncompensated elasticities of demand from the GODDS model

				With respect to price of				
Elasticity of demand for	Cereals and bakery	Meat and eggs	Dairy	Fruits and vegetables	Non-alcoholic drinks	Other FAH	FAFH and alcohol	Nonfood
Cereals and bakery	-0.58	0.05	0.36	-0.31	-0.09	0.25	0.16	0.16
	(0.25)	(0.12)	(0.08)	(0.13)	(0.15)	(0.29)	(0.34)	(0.29)
Meat and eggs	0.03	-0.31	0.02	0.11	0.08	0.26	0.17	-0.40
	(0.07)	(0.17)	(0.05)	(0.09)	(0.04)	(0.11)	(0.32)	(0.40)
Dairy	0.49	0.06	-0.05	-0.03	-0.16	-0.44	0.23	-0.21
	(0.10)	(0.12)	(0.09)	(0.11)	(0.07)	(0.16)	(0.30)	(0.29)
Fruits and vegetables	-0.30	0.18	-0.02	-0.79	0.02	0.58	0.24	0.04
	(0.13)	(0.15)	(0.08)	(0.19)	(0.09)	(0.20)	(0.39)	(0.36)
Nonalcoholic beverages	-0.21	0.31	-0.25	0.05	-0.65	0.65	-0.05	0.13
	(0.32)	(0.16)	(0.12)	(0.20)	(0.39)	(0.46)	(0.51)	(0.38)
Other FAH	0.15	0.27	-0.19	0.36	0.18	-0.98	0.45	-0.32
	(0.18)	(0.11)	(0.07)	(0.12)	(0.12)	(0.30)	(0.34)	(0.28)
FAFH and alcohol	0.03	0.05	0.03	0.05	-0.01	0.14	-0.71	0.20
	(0.07)	(0.11)	(0.04)	(0.08)	(0.05)	(0.11)	(0.38)	(0.37)
Nonfood	-0.02	-0.05	-0.02	-0.02	-0.01	-0.04	-0.06	-1.00
	(0.01)	(0.01)	(0.00)	(0.01)	(0.00)	(0.01)	(0.04)	(0.06)

Elasticity of demand for	With respect to total expenditure	R^2	Breusch-Godfrey statistic	Constant
Cereals and bakery	0.01	0.77	1.66	0.0002
	(0.05)			(0.0001)
Meat and eggs	0.04	0.59	4.90	0.0005
	(0.07)			(0.0002)
Dairy	0.11			0.0001
	(0.05)	0.74	2.20	(0.0001)
Fruits and vegetables	0.04	0.66	5.87	-0.0002
	(0.06)			(0.0001)
Nonalcoholic beverages	0.02	0.70	0.18	0.0000
	(0.05)			(0.0001)
Other FAH	0.09	0.76	0.08	-0.0003
	(0.04)			(0.0002)
FAFH and alcohol	0.21	0.58	3.63	0.0003
	(0.06)			
Nonfood	1.21			
	(0.01)	na	na	na

Source: Authors' calculations using feasible generalized least squares GLS (Stata version 11) with homogeneity and symmetry constraints imposed.

Notes: Estimates of elasticities of demand were computed at the mean of the data. Standard errors were bootstrapped using the residual method. Total expenditure includes expenditures on durable and nondurable goods and services. The R^2 and the Breusch-Godfrey statistic are for the individual equations and Breusch-Godfrey statistic is distributed $\chi^2(1)$, for which the 10% critical value is 2.71.

FAFH = Food away from home, including limited-service and full-service restaurants; FAH = Food at home; GODDS = Generalized Ordinary Differential Demand System.

Table 5. Comparison of first-stage elasticities of demand from this study with previous studies

	This study		Reed, Levedahl, Hallahan (2005)		Huang and Lin (2000)[b]		Park et al. (1996)[c]		Okrent and Alston (2011), table 5	
	Own-price	Expen-diture	Own-price	Income	Own-price	Expen-diture	Own-price	Expen-diture	Number of studies represented	Average own-price across studies
Cereals and bakery	-0.58	0.01	-0.61	1.31	-0.45	0.63	-0.14	0.43	3	-0.86
Meat and eggs	-0.31	0.04	-0.61	1.81	-0.41	0.78	-0.45	0.64	8	-0.52
Dairy	-0.05	0.11	-0.86	2.25	-0.79	0.67	-0.36	0.57	8	-0.85
Fruits and vegetables	-0.79	0.04	-0.98	1.60	-0.72	1.07	-0.49	0.65	4	-0.91
Nonalcoholic beverages	-0.65	0.02	-0.74[a]	1.04a	-1.01	1.04	na	na	na	na
Other FAH	-0.98	0.09			-0.40	0.82	-0.58	0.59	11	-0.80
FAFH and alcohol	-0.71	0.21	-0.69	1.38	na	na	-0.96	1.42	8	-1.02
Nonfood	-1.00	1.21	-0.86	0.92	na	na	na	na	2	-0.93

Source: Estimates for this study based on the GODDS and average monthly household expenditures based on the Consumer Expenditure Survey (U.S. Department of Labor, BLS, 2010a) and the Consumer Price Indexes (U.S. Department of Labor, BLS, 2010c).

a Nonalcoholic beverages included in other FAH category.

b The own-price and expenditure elasticities in this table are simple averages for disaggregated elasticities presented in Huang and Lin (2000) within the groups comprising cereals and bakery, meat and eggs, dairy, and fruits and vegetables.

c Estimates for nonpoverty status households only (table 8). The own-price and expenditure elasticities in this table are simple averages for disaggregated elasticities presented in Park et al. (1996) within the groups comprising cereals and bakery, meat and eggs, dairy, and fruits/ vegetables. The other FAH category only includes fats and oils.

FAFH = Food away from home, including limited-service and full-service restaurants; FAH = Food-at-home; GODDS = Generalized Ordinary Differential Demand System.

Demand for nonfood is found to be the most responsive to changes in own price (own-price elasticity of -1.00), followed by other FAH (own-price elasticity of -0.98). The own-price elasticity of demand for FAFH and alcohol is -0.71, which compares well with the estimate by Reed, Levedahl, and Hallahan (2005), but is considerably less than in other studies. Okrent and Alston (2011) found that across eight studies the average of the estimates of own-price elasticity of demand for FAFH was -1.02 (table 5). In fact, all of this study's own-price elasticities are less than the average across studies reported in Okrent and Alston (2011). Our first-stage own-price elasticities are mostly consistent with those of Reed, Levedahl, and Hallahan (2005); Huang and Lin (2000); and Park et al. (1996). Of the 56 cross-price elasticities of demand, 20 are statistically significant at the 10-percent level of significance. Many of the FAH products (i.e., cereals and bakery products, dairy, and other FAH) are gross substitutes for FAFH and alcohol, although these relationships are not found to be statistically significant. Other FAH is a statistically significant gross substitute for both meat/eggs and fruits/vegetables, but a gross complement for dairy. And dairy is also found to be a statistically significant gross complement for nonalcoholic beverages. Not unexpectedly, demand for nonfood is the most responsive to total expenditure (elasticity of 1.21), followed by demand for FAFH and alcohol (0.21). Demands for FAFH and alcohol are twice as responsive to changes in total expenditure as the most expenditure-elastic FAH products, namely dairy (0.11) and other FAH (0.09). Compared with the total-expenditure elasticities from the studies listed in table 5, the ones here are quite small, mainly because the nonfood budget share is 80 percent.

Conditional Elasticities of Demand for Disaggregated Food Products

We estimated demand for disaggregated food products, assuming the products belonged to the following weakly separable groups: cereals and bakery products, meat and eggs, dairy products, fruits and vegetables, nonalcoholic beverages, other FAH, and FAFH/alcohol. Hence, the elasticities of demand for the disaggregated FAH products are conditional on total expenditure for the respective group. First-order autocorrelation is not detected in most of the second-stage estimates, with the exception of nonalcoholic beverages, based on the Rao-Breusch-Godfrey test. The system R^2 for the second-stage allocations ranges between 0.07 for other FAH and cereals/bakery products and 0.20 for dairy. For brevity, we report the elasticities of demand, single-equation R^2, first-order autocorrelation coefficient, Breusch-Godfrey LM statistic, and the trend term in each equation for the second-stage allocations in appendix tables A.3-A.9.

Unconditional Elasticities of Demand for Disaggregated Food Products

Using equations (11) and (12) and the estimated elasticities of demand from the models of the first- and second-stage allocations, we approximated the elasticities of demand for disaggregated FAH and FAFH products conditional on total expenditure for all goods and services. Table 6 shows the own-price and expenditure elasticities of demand for disaggregated food products compared with Huang (1993) and Bergtold, Akobundo, and Peterson (2004).[12] Appendix table A.10. contains the 43 × 43 matrix of all elasticities. The standard errors were bootstrapped using the parametric residual method suggested by Green, Hahn, and Rocke (1987).

Cereals and Bakery Products

The demands for flour and prepared flour mixes; rice and pasta; and biscuits, rolls, and muffins are almost perfectly inelastic; the point estimates are close to zero and not statistically significantly different from zero (table 6). These findings approximate those of Huang (1993). By comparison, Bergtold, Akobundu, and Peterson (2004) found the own-price elasticity of demand to be closer to -1.0 for rice, pasta, and flour, but only the own-price elasticity of demand for pasta was statistically significant. The demands for breakfast cereals and cakes/cookies are price-elastic (i.e., elasticities of -1.05 and -1.20, respectively).

The demand for nonwhite bread is less responsive to changes in price than the demand for white bread (elasticities of -0.59 and -1.54, respectively). Most of the cross-price elasticities of demand for foods within the cereals and bakery products group are statistically insignificant, although white bread and nonwhite bread are statistically significant gross substitutes, and flour/prepared flour mixes is a gross substitute for rice and pasta and a gross complement to nonwhite bread.

Compared with the disaggregated demands of the other groups, the demands for all of the cereals and bakery products are relatively expenditure-inelastic, with elasticities ranging between 0.00 and 0.01. Bergtold, Akobundu, and Peterson (2004) and Huang (1993) also found the demands for disaggregated cereals and bakery products to be expenditure-inelastic and even inferior (i.e., expenditure elasticity is less than zero), compared to disaggregated products within other food groups.

Meat and Eggs

Pork and "other red meat" (that is, other than beef and pork) are price-elastic (own-price elasticities of -1.26 and -1.05), while the other products in the meat and eggs group—beef, poultry, fish/seafood, and eggs—are price inelastic, with eggs being the most price inelastic (own-price elasticity of -0.24).

The rankings of meat products in terms of their price responsiveness are roughly consistent with results from Huang (1993), although some of our estimates are statistically significantly smaller, at the 10-percent level of significance (e.g., pork, other red meat, fish/seafood, and eggs). Also, similar to Huang's findings (1993), beef and pork are statistically significant gross substitutes for each another.

Demands for meat products are slightly more responsive to changes in total expenditure than are demands for cereals and bakery products, with expenditure elasticities ranging between 0.02 for other red meat and 0.05 for beef. But this effect is still small and insignificant compared to the other products in the system.

Table 6. Comparison of unconditional elasticities of demand from this study with previous studies

	This study		Bergtold, Akobundu, and Peterson (2004)[a,b]		Huang (1993)[b]	
	Own-price	Expenditure	Own-price	Income	Own-price	Expenditure
Cereals and bakery						
Flour and flour mixes	0.07	0.01	-0.86	0.06	-0.08	0.13
Breakfast cereals	-1.05*	0.00	na	na	na	0
Rice and pasta	-0.07	0.01	-0.87	-0.06	0.07	0.15
Nonwhite bread	-0.59*	0.00	-0.80	-0.21	na	na
White bread	-1.54	0.01			na	na
Biscuits, rolls, muffins	-0.21	0.00	-1.03	-0.55	na	na
Cakes and cookies	-1.20*	0.01	na	na	na	na
Other bakery products	-0.55	0.00	na	na	na	na
Meat and eggs						
Beef	-0.70*	0.05	na	na	-0.62	0.39

Table 6. (Continued)

	This study		Bergtold, Akobundu, and Peterson (2004)[a,b]		Huang (1993)[b]	
	Own-price	Expenditure	Own-price	Income	Own-price	Expenditure
Pork	-1.26*	0.04	na	na	-0.73	0.66
Other red meat	-1.05*	0.02	na	na	-1.87	-0.57
Poultry	-0.81*	0.03	na	na	-0.45	-0.02
Fish	-0.84*	0.03	na	na	-0.13	0.41
Eggs	-0.24*	0.03	na	na	-0.11	0.29
Dairy						
Cheese	-0.70*	0.13*	-1.18	-0.03	-0.25	0.42
Ice cream	-0.23	0.13*	-0.88	0.05	-0.08	0.00
Milk	-0.10	0.09*	-0.80	-0.20	-0.04	0.12
Other dairy	-1.04*	0.09*	-1.03	0.31	-0.28	0.52
Fruits and vegetables						
Apples	-0.58*	0.03	na	na	-0.19	-0.36
Bananas	-1.01*	0.05	na	na	-0.50	0.00
Citrus	-1.10*	0.06	na	na	-0.65	-0.33
Other fresh fruit	-0.90*	0.04	na	na	-0.80	0.34
Potatoes	-0.42*	0.03	na	na	-0.10	0.11
Lettuce	-0.84*	0.04	na	na	-0.09	0.37
Tomatoes	-0.58*	0.06	na	na	-0.62	0.92
Other fresh vegetables	-0.94*	0.04	na	na	-0.26	0.69
Proc. fruits and vegetables	-0.77*	0.03	-1.20	-0.29	-0.40	0.56
Nonalcoholic beverages						
Coffee and tea	-0.12	0.02	-0.45	-0.27	-0.18	0.82
Carbonated drinks	-0.30	0.01	-1.15	-0.03	na	na
Nonfrozen noncarb. drinks	-0.44	0.02	-0.65	-0.12	-0.56	0.37
Frozen noncarb. drinks	-0.61	0.01	-0.70	-0.14	na	na
Other food at home						
Sugar and sweets	-0.56	0.13*	-0.66	-0.16	-0.04	0.21
Fats and oils	-0.21	0.08*	-0.62	-0.51	-0.13	0.23
Soups	0.19*	0.07*	-1.51	0.59	na	na
Frozen foods	-1.05	0.09*	-1.08	-0.27	na	na
Snacks	-1.14*	0.08*	-1.17	-0.10	na	na
Condiments, sauces, seas.	-1.92*	0.07*	-1.00	-0.01	na	na
Misc. FAH	-1.48*	0.11*	-1.17	0.01	na	na
Food away from home/alcohol						
Alcohol	-1.15*	0.32*	na	na	na	na

	This study		Bergtold, Akobundu, and Peterson (2004)[a,b]		Huang (1993)[b]	
	Own-price	Expenditure	Own-price	Income	Own-price	Expenditure
Limited-service	-0.13	0.18*	Na	na	na	na
Full-service	-1.96*	0.20*	na	na	na	na
Other FAFH	-0.43*	0.21*	na	na	na	na
Nonfood	-1.00*	1.21*	-1.00	0.99	-0.98	1.17

* designates statistical significance at the 10-percent level for estimates in this study only.

a Bergtold et al. (2004) presented own-price and expenditure elasticities of demand for four quarters. We averaged the elasticity estimates over the quarters.

b Some of the products in Bergtold et al. (2004) and Huang (1993) did not correspond directly to the products in this study. Hence, we calculated the average own-price and expenditure elasticities of demand for multiple products that corresponded to a product in this study. Source: Estimates from this study based on first-stage elasticities of demand (table 4), second-stage elasticities of demand (appendix tables A.4-A.9) and formulas derived by Carpentier and Guyomard (2001) in equations (12) and (13).

FAFH = Food away from home, including limited-service and full-service restaurants; FAH = Food-at-home.

Dairy

The own-price elasticities of demand for cheese and other dairy are statistically different from zero at the 10-percent level of significance (-0.70 and -1.04, respectively) and much more price-elastic than the demands for fluid milk and ice cream/frozen desserts (-0.10 and -0.23, respectively), which are not found to be statistically significant. Huang (1993) found demand for similar dairy products to be mostly price-inelastic, whereas Bergtold, Akobundu, and Peterson (2004) found demand for comparable items to be much more elastic. Our results fall between the two studies' findings. Cheese is found to be a statistically significant gross substitute for other dairy, which includes yogurt and sour cream. Compared with the disaggregated demands in the cereals/bakery, meat/eggs, fruits/vegetables, and nonalcoholic beverages groups, demands for disaggregated dairy products are almost twice as responsive to changes in total expenditure, with expenditure elasticities ranging between 0.09 for milk and other dairy and 0.13 for cheese and ice cream. Again, these estimated elasticities of demand with respect to total expenditure fall generally in between the estimates of Bergtold, Akobundu, and Peterson (2004) and Huang (1993). Bergtold, Akobundu, and Peterson found cheese and milk to be inferior products (a good that decreases in demand when income increases) and the elasticity of demand for ice cream and cheese with respect to total expenditure to be close to zero.

Fruits and Vegetables

In this group, all of the own-price elasticities are statistically significant, with demand for citrus being the most elastic (own-price elasticity of -1.10) and demand for potatoes being the least elastic (own-price elasticity of -0.42). Within the fruits and vegetables group, few of the cross-price relationships are statistically significant with the exception of processed fruits and vegetables, which is a gross complement to fresh tomatoes. The elasticities of demand for the disaggregated fruits and vegetables with respect to total expenditure are small, ranging between 0.03 and 0.06. Compared with Huang (1993), the present study finds the demands for disaggregated fruits and vegetables to be generally more price-elastic and more expenditure-inelastic.

Nonalcoholic Beverages

Within this group, none of the elasticities of demand with respect to price or expenditure elasticities is significant. The elasticities of demand with respect to total expenditure are close to zero, and the own-price elasticities of demand are small compared with most other food products, with the demand for coffee and tea being the least price responsive at -0.12. Huang (1993) found the own-price elasticity of demand for coffee and tea to be -0.18, while Bergtold, Akobundu, and Peterson (2004) found the own-price elasticity for coffee to be -0.45. However, Bergtold, Akobundu, and Peterson (2004) found the demand for carbonated beverages (averaged across diet and regular cola estimates) to be much more price elastic (-1.15) than our estimate for carbonated beverages (-0.30).

Other FAH

Most of the demands for products within the other FAH group are price-elastic, with seasonings, condiments, and sauces being the most price elastic (-1.92), followed by miscellaneous FAH (-1.48), snacks (-1.14), and frozen meals (-1.05). This finding is consistent with Bergtold, Akobundu and Peterson (2004), who found sauces and marinades, mayonnaise, relishes, and dressings to be generally price elastic. We find the demands for sugars/ sweets and fats/oils to be price-inelastic, but both relationships are statistically insignificant. Compared with the other food product categories, the "other FAH" products are the most responsive to changes in their own price with the exception of FAFH and alcohol.

FAFH and Alcohol

The demands for limited-service FAFH and other FAFH (vending machines, mobile food vendors, and school/employee sites) are the most inelastic in the group (-0.13 and -0.43, respectively). The own-price elasticity of demand for full-service FAFH is -1.96, and is statistically different from the own-price elasticity of demand for limited-service FAFH at the 10-percent level of significance.

Full- and limited-service FAFH are found to be gross substitutes, although this relationship is not statistically significant. Demand for alcohol is also price-elastic (-1.15).

All of the FAFH products and alcohol are more than twice as responsive to changes in total expenditure compared to the FAH products. Alcohol is the most price-responsive (0.32), followed by other FAFH (0.21), full-service FAFH (0.20), and limited-service FAFH (0.18).

POTENTIAL POLICY IMPLICATIONS

Because disaggregated FAFH and FAH products may differ in responsiveness to prices and total expenditure, as well as in nutritional content, we estimate elasticities using a more disaggregated approach than previously done in the literature.

Our results show that the demand for full-service FAFH is much more responsive than the demand for limited-service FAFH to changes in price, and the demands for all FAFH products are at least twice as elastic with respect to changes in total expenditure than their FAH counterparts. The finding that FAFH products are much more responsive to changes in total expenditure—and that these FAFH products are generally gross substitutes for many FAH products—can explain why the budget share for these products dipped during the 2007-09 recession, while the budget shares for many FAH products increased.

In particular, during the period of December 2007- June 2009, monthly total consumer expenditures fell by about 0.5 percent on average, while the prices of most FAH products, which are mostly gross substitutes for FAFH products, fell relative to the prices of the FAFH products. Hence, income-induced changes in total expenditures and movements in prices of FAH products relative to prices of FAFH products caused demand for FAFH to fall during the most recent recession.

The demands for disaggregated FAH products, which include some foods that are considered to be "healthy" and others considered too be "unhealthy," also varied in their responsiveness to changes in prices and total expenditure. "Healthy" foods—such as nonwhite bread, most fruits and vegetables, and fish/seafood—are generally less responsive to changes in their own prices than their "unhealthy" counterparts.

For example, for cereals and bakery products, we found that the unconditional demand for white bread was much more price elastic than the unconditional demand for nonwhite bread, and the demand for cookies and cakes was one of the most price elastic within the group. Likewise, the unconditional demands for snacks, condiments/sauces/ seasonings, and frozen foods were very price elastic compared with the demands for other FAH products.

However, own-price effects are only one part of an analysis of the effects of policy-induced price changes on consumption. The cross-price relationships between "unhealthy" and "healthy" foods are complex; in analyzing the effect of a change in the price of a "healthy" or "unhealthy" food on the nutritional outcome of an individual, one must consider the cross-price, as well as the own-price, effects.

To further demonstrate the importance of these cross-price relationships and intergroup substitution on the quantities of food consumed, we forecast the changes in consumption for several foods between 2011 and 2012— given forecast changes in prices and total expenditures—and compare the predictions based on alternative elasticity measures. We use the "unconditional" demand elasticities reported in appendix table A.10 to obtain forecasts that consider intergroup as well as intragroup substitution; and we use the "conditional" demand elasticities reported in appendix tables A.3-A.9 (i.e., conditional on group expenditure) to obtain forecasts that consider only intragroup substitution.

The forecast changes in prices of food from 2011 to 2012 are taken from the CPI forecasts by the U.S. Department of Agriculture, ERS (2011), and the forecast changes in prices for nonfood and total expenditures are taken from the Federal Reserve Bank of Philadelphia's Fourth Quarter 2011 Survey of Professional Forecasters (2011) (table 7).[13]

According to the ERS price forecasts, the prices of beef, fish/seafood, fats/oils, and cereals/bakery products will increase the most (between 4 and 4.5 percent) from 2011 to 2012, whereas the prices for fresh vegetables, eggs, and nonalcoholic beverages will increase the least, between 1.5 and 2 percent. The price of nonfood products, as proxied by core inflation for 2012, is predicted to increase by 1.8 percent, while total personal consumption expenditures are predicted to increase 1.7 percent.

Using these predicted changes in prices and total expenditure, we forecast changes in food quantities using both unconditional and conditional elasticities. Both sets of forecasts indicate decreases in the quantities of disaggregated cereals and bakery products consumed, but the magnitudes differ substantially; the forecasts based on the conditional elasticities of demand are three to four times larger in absolute terms than the forecasts based on the unconditional elasticities of demand.

Even though the conditional own-price elasticities of demand were not statistically different from the unconditional own-price elasticities of demand at the 10-percent level of significance, the conditional forecasts disregarded statistically significant intergroup substitution and complementary relationships found in the first stage (i.e., dairy, fruits/vegetables, and nonfood). The conditional forecasts followed the same pattern for the disaggregated FAFH products.

The predicted percentage changes in dairy consumption based on the elasticities of demand conditional on dairy expenditure take opposite signs compared with the predicted percentage changes based on the unconditional elasticities of demand: consumption of each of the disaggregated dairy products is predicted to *increase* between 0.61 percent and 0.9 percent in 2012 based on the unconditional demand elasticities, but predicted to *decrease* between 0.63 percent and 0.97 percent based on the conditional demand elasticities. Similar contradictions between the two sets of elasticities are found for other food products as well (e.g., pork, poultry, eggs, sugar and sweets, frozen foods). Again, dairy—like cereals and bakery products—has several statistically significant cross-price relationships between groups of foods at the first stage that results in complementary and substitution relationships among the disaggregated products in these groups, causing contradictions in our forecast changes in quantities consumed depending on which set of elasticities is used.

The substantial cross-price relationships between products in different groups lead to two important and related implications. First, the predicted changes in quantities of foods consumed based on the conditional demand elasticities pertaining to a weakly separable group are different in magnitude, and sometimes in direction of change, than predicted changes in quantities based on unconditional elasticities of demand. Second, policy analysis based on conditional demand elasticities for a small group of products is likely to be misleading.

Table 7. Forecast changes in food consumption, 2011 to 2012, based on forecast changes in prices and expenditure, using alternative sets of elasticities of demand

	Forecast changes in prices and total expenditure	Predicted changes in food quantities based on		Predicted changes in expenditures based on	
		Unconditional elasticities[a]	Conditional elasticities[b]	Unconditional elasticities[a]	Conditional elasticities[b]
Flour and prep. mixes	4.0	-1.25	-4.23	2.75	-0.23
Breakfast cereals	4.0	-0.48	-1.56	3.52	2.44
Rice and pasta	4.0	-1.01	-3.69	2.99	0.31
Nonwhite bread	4.0	-0.44	-1.62	3.56	2.38
White bread	4.0	-0.78	-2.63	3.22	1.37
Biscuits, rolls, muffins	4.0	-0.39	-1.81	3.61	2.19
Cakes and cookies	4.0	-0.84	-2.67	3.16	1.33
Other bakery	4.0	-0.55	-1.92	3.45	2.09
Beef	4.5	-0.39	-3.39	4.11	1.11
Pork	3.5	0.58	-1.75	4.08	1.75
Other red meat	3.0	1.35	0.07	4.35	3.07
Poultry	3.5	0.28	-1.31	3.78	2.19
Fish	4.5	-1.08	-3.11	3.43	1.39
Eggs	1.5	0.75	-0.77	2.25	0.73
Cheese	2.5	0.90	-0.97	3.40	1.53
Ice cream and frozen desserts	2.5	0.87	-0.92	3.37	1.58
Milk	2.5	0.61	-0.63	3.11	1.87
Other dairy	2.5	0.69	-0.71	3.19	1.80
Apples	3.5	-0.70	-1.55	2.81	1.95
Bananas	3.5	-0.62	-2.11	2.88	1.39
Citrus	3.5	-0.91	-2.64	2.59	0.86
Other fruits	3.5	-0.16	-1.45	3.35	2.05
Potatoes	1.5	0.90	0.09	2.40	1.59
Lettuce	1.5	1.02	-0.38	2.52	1.12
Tomatoes	1.5	0.22	-1.55	1.72	-0.05
Other veg.	1.5	1.66	0.27	3.16	1.77
Processed fruits/vegetables	3.5	-0.32	-1.15	3.18	2.35
Coffee and tea	2.0	0.78	-0.16	2.78	1.84
Carbonated drinks	2.0	0.66	-0.31	2.66	1.69
Nonfrozen noncarbonated drinks	2.0	1.06	-0.35	3.06	1.65
Frozen noncarbonated drinks	2.0	0.44	-0.22	2.44	1.78
Sugar and sweets	2.5	0.56	-2.06	3.06	0.44
Fats and oils	4.0	-0.07	-1.62	3.93	2.38
Soups	3.5	1.86	1.00	5.36	4.50
Frozen foods	3.5	0.63	-1.15	4.14	2.35
Snacks	3.5	-0.08	-1.59	3.42	1.91
Condiments, sauces, seasonings	3.5	-0.80	-2.20	2.70	1.30
Misc. food at home	3.5	-0.13	-2.28	3.37	1.22

	Forecast changes in prices and total expenditure	Predicted changes in food quantities based on		Predicted changes in expenditures based on	
		Unconditional elasticities[a]	Conditional elasticities[b]	Unconditional elasticities[a]	Conditional elasticities[b]
Alcohol	3.0	-0.61	-1.93	2.39	1.07
Limited	3.0	-0.42	-1.09	2.58	1.91
Full	3.0	-0.49	-1.22	2.51	1.78
Other food away from home	3.0	-0.51	-1.30	2.49	1.70
Nonfood	1.8	-0.35	na	1.45	na

Notes: Forecast changes in food prices from 2011 to 2012 are based on forecast changes in Consumer Price Index for foods (U.S. Department of Agriculture, ERS, 2011); forecast changes in the nonfood price and total expenditure are based on the mean of reported predictions for 2012 by a sample of professional forecasters for core inflation and headline personal consumption expenditures (Federal Reserve Board of Philadelphia, 2011).

[a] The predictions based on the unconditional elasticities of demand use elasticities of demand reported in appendix table A.10.

[b] The predictions based on conditional elasticities of demand use elasticities reported in appendix tables A.3-A.9.

CONCLUSION

Many studies have evaluated the effect of policy-induced price changes on food consumption and nutritional outcomes. Several studies have based their analysis on demand elasticities for only a subset of foods (i.e., conditional on expenditure for a particular group of foods), which ignores important cross-price relationships of foods not included in a given analysis. In particular, because FAFH comprises a significant share of total food expenditures and nutritional intake for an average American, disregarding the potential cross-price relationship between FAFH and another relevant subset of foods may lead to misleading results regarding nutrition and health policy. This study is the first to present disaggregated estimates of demand elasticities for different types of FAFH within a complete demand system for food, alcohol, and nonfood. We find that the demand for full-service FAFH is much more price-elastic than the demand for food from limited-service restaurants. All of the disaggregated products within FAFH are much more responsive to changes in total expenditure than all of the FAH products. Hence, our findings suggest that decreases in total expenditure during the most recent recession had a much greater impact on demands for most FAFH products than for FAH products. We also present disaggregated elasticities of demand for FAH products. The demands for products within any group can vary considerably in terms of responsiveness to price changes, aggregating groups in policy simulations masks important dissimilarities within food groups in terms of nutrient characteristics and responses to prices and total expenditure. In particular, the demands for products commonly deemed to be "healthy" (fruits and vegetables, nonwhite bread, fish and seafood) tend to be much less responsive to own-price changes compared with those commonly deemed to be "unhealthy" (e.g., white bread, cakes and cookies, frozen foods, snacks). Many of these "healthy" and "unhealthy" foods are found to have statistically significant substitution and complementary relationships within and among food groups, which complicates analysis that tries to predict the effects of policy-induced changes in prices and income on demands for foods and the nutritional outcomes of consumers. Consequently, forecasts of the changes of quantities of food based on estimates of conditional demand elasticities that ignore the total effects of intergroup substitution and complementarities differ substantially in magnitude and sometimes even direction from forecasts based on estimates of unconditional demand elasticities that include all goods and services.

REFERENCES

Andreyeva, T., M.W. Long, and K.D. Brownell. 2009. "The Impact of Food Prices on Consumption: A Systematic Review of Research on the Price Elasticity of Demand for Food," *American Journal of Public Health* 100(2): 216-222.

Barnes, R., and R. Gillingham. 1984. "Demographic Effects in Demand Analysis: Estimation of the Quadratic Expenditure System Using Microdata," *The Review of Economics and Statistics* 66(4): 591-601.

Barten, A.P. 1966. "Theorie en empirie van een volledig stelsel van vraagvergelijkiingrn," Doctoral dissertation: University of Rotterdam.

Barten, A.P. 1969. "Maximum Likelihood Estimation of a Complete System of Demand Equations," *European Economic Review* 1: 7-73.

Barten, A.P. 1977. "The Systems of Consumer Demand Functions Approach: A Review." *Econometrica* 45): 23-50.

Barten, A.P. 1993. "Consumer Allocation Models: Choice of Functional Form." *Empirical Economics* 18(1):129-158.

Beaulieu, J.J., and J.A. Miron. 1993. "Seasonal Unit Roots in Aggregate U.S. Data," *Journal of Econometrics* 55(1/2): 305-328.

Bergtold, J., E. Akobundu, and E. Peterson. 2004. "The FAST Method: Estimating Unconditional Demand Elasticities for Processed Foods in the Presence of Fixed Effects," *Journal of Agricultural and Resource Economics* 29(2): 276-295.

Berndt, E.R., and N.E. Savin. 1975. "Estimation and Hypothesis Testing in Singular Equation Systems with Autoregressive Disturbances," *Econometrica* 43(5/6): 937-958.

Bewley, R., T. Young, and D. Colman. 1987. "A System Approach to Modeling Supply Equations in Agriculture," *Journal of Agricultural Economics* 38(2): 151-66.

Binkley, J.K. 2008. "Calorie and Gram Differences between Meals at Fast Food and Table Service Restaurants," *Review of Agricultural Economics* 30(4): 750-763.

Brown, M.G., J.Y. Lee, and J.L. Seale. 1994. "Demand Relationships among Juice Beverages: A Differential Demand System Approach," *Journal of Agricultural and Applied Economics* 26: 417-417.

Byrne, P.J., O. Capps, and A. Saha. 2008. "Analysis of Quick-serve, Mid-scale, and Up-scale Food Away from Home Expenditures," *International Food and Agribusiness Management Review* 1(1): 51-72.

Capps, O., and J. Havlicek. 1984. "National and Regional Household Demand for Meat, Poultry and Seafood: A Complete Systems Approach," *Canadian Journal of Agricultural Economics* 32(1): 93-108.

Carpentier, A., and H. Guyomard. "Unconditional Elasticities in Two-Stage Systems: An Approximate Solution," *American Journal of Agricultural Economics* 83(1): 222-229.

Chen, S.E., R.J.G.M. Florax, and S.D. Snyder. *Forthcoming.* "Obesity and Fast-Food Markets: A New Approach Using Geo-referenced Micro Data." *Health Economics*.

Chou, S.-Y., M. Grossman, and H. Saffer. 2004. "An economic analysis of adult obesity: results from the Behavioral Risk Factor Surveillance System," *Journal of Health Economics* 23(3): 565-587.

Christensen, L.R., D.W. Jorgenson, and L.J. Lau. 1975. "Transcendental Logarithmic Utility Functions," *American Economic Review* 65: 367-83.

Craven, J.A. and R.C. Haidacher. 1987. "Comparison of Estimates from Three Linear Expenditure Systems," *Food Demand Analysis: Problems, Issues, and Empirical Evidence*. R. Raunikar and C. Huang, editors. Iowa State University Press, 91-113.

Currie, J., S. Della Vigna, E. Moretti, and V. Pathania. 2010. "The Effect of Fast Food Restaurants on Obesity and Weight Gain," *American Economic Journal: Economic Policy* (2)(3): 32-63.

Davis, B., and C. Carpenter. 2009. "Proximity of Fast-Food Restaurants to Schools and Adolescent Obesity," *American Journal of Public Health* 99(3): 505-510.

Deaton, A., and J. Muellbauer. 1980a. "An Almost Ideal Demand System," *The American Economic Review* 70(3): 312-326.

Deaton, A., and J. Muellbauer.1980b. *Economics and Consumer Behavior*. New York, NY: Cambridge University Press.

Eales, J., C. Durham, and C.R. Wessells. 1997. "Generalized Models of Japanese Demand for Fish," *American Journal of Agricultural Economics* 79(4): 1153-1163.

Edgarton, D.L., and G. Shukur. 1999. "Testing Autocorrelation in a System Perspective," *Econometric Reviews* 18: 343-86.

Federal Reserve Board of Philadelphia. 2011. Fourth Quarter 2011 Survey of Professional Forecasters, Nov. 14, 2011. http://www.philadelphiafed.org/research-and-data/real-time-center/survey-of-professional-forecasters/2011/survq411.cfm.

Gao, X.M., and J.S. Shonkwiler. 1993. "Characterizing Taste Change in a Model of US Meat Demand: Correcting for Spurious Regression and Measurement Errors," *Review of Agricultural Economics* 15(2): 313-324.

Gao, X.M., and T. Spreen. 1994. "A Microeconometric Analysis of the US Meat Demand," *Canadian Journal of Agricultural Economics* 42(3): 397-412.

Gorman, W.M. 1959. "Separable Utility and Aggregation," *Econometrica* 27(3) :469-481.

Green, R., W. Hahn, and D. Rocke. 1987. "Standard Errors for Elasticities: A Comparison of Bootstrap and Asymptotic Standard Errors," *Journal of Business and Economic Statistics* 5(1): 145-149.

Greene, W.H. 2003. *Econometric Analysis*, 5th ed. New York: Prentice Hall, Inc.

Heien, D.M., and G. Pompelli. 1988. "The Demand for Beef Products: Cross-Section Estimation of Demographic and Economic Effects," *Western Journal of Agricultural Economics* 13(1): 37-44.

Huang, K.S. 1993. *A Complete System of U.S. Demand for Food*. TB-1821. USDA, Economic Research Service.

Huang, K.S., and B.-H. Lin.2000. *Estimation of Food Demand and Nutrient Elasticities from Household Survey Data.* TB-1887. USDA, Economic Research Service.

Hylleberg, S., R.F. Engle, C.W.S Granger, and B.S. Yoo. 1990. "Seasonal Integration and Cointegration," *Journal of Econometrics* 44: 215-238.

Jeffrey, R.W., J. Baxter, M. McGuire, J. Linde. "Are Fast-Food Restaurants an Environmental Risk Factor for Obesity?" *International Journal of Behavior Nutrition and Physical Activity* 3(2)(2006).

Kastens, T.L., and G.W. Brester. 1996. "Model Selection and Forecasting Ability of Theory-Constrained Food Demand Systems," *American Journal of Agricultural Economics* 78(2): 301-312.

Keller, W.J., and J. Van Driel. 1985. "Differential Consumer Demand Systems," *European Economic Review* 27(3): 375-390.

Kmenta, J., and R.F. Gilbert. 1968. "Small Sample Properties of Alternative Estimators of Seemingly Unrelated Regressions," *Journal of the American Statistical Association* 63: 1180-1200.

Lee, J.Y., M.G. Brown, and J.L. Seale. "Model Choice in Consumer Analysis: Taiwan, 1970-1989," *American Journal of Agricultural Economics* 76(3): 504-512.

Leser, C.E.V. 1963. "Forms of Engel Functions," *Econometrica* 31(4): 694-703.

Lin, B.-H., J. Guthrie, and E. Frazao. 1999. *Away-From-Home Foods Increasingly Important to Quality of American Diet.* AIB-749. U.S. Department of Agriculture, Economic Research Service.

Matsuda, T. 2005. "Differential Demand Systems: A Further Look at Barten's Synthesis," *Southern Economic Journal* 71(3): 607-619.

Moschini, G. 1998. "The Semiflexible Almost Ideal Demand System," *European Economic Review* (42): 349-364.

Moschini, G. 2001. "A Flexible Multistage Demand System Based on Indirect Separability." *Southern Economic* Journal 68(1): 22-41.

Nayga, R.M., and O. Capps.1992. "Analysis of Food Away from Home and Food at Home Consumption: A Systems Approach," *Journal of Food Distribution Research* 23(6).

Neves, P. 1987. "Analysis of Consumer Demand in Portugal, 1958-1981." *Memorie de Maitrise en Sciences Economiques.* Louvain-la-Neuve, France: University Catholiqque de Louvrain.

Okrent, A.M., and J.M. Alston. 2011. *The Demand for Food in the United States: A Review of the Literature, Evaluation of Previous Estimates, and Presentation of New Estimates of Demand.* Giannini Foundation of Agricultural Economics Monograph 48, Berkeley, CA, April.

Park, J.L., R.B. Holcomb, K.C. Raper, and O. Capps.1996. "A Demand Systems Analysis of Food Commodities by U.S. Households Segmented by Income," *American Journal of Agricultural Economics* 78(2): 290-300.

Piggott, N.E. 2003. "The Nested PIGLOG Model: An Application to US Food Demand." *American Journal of Agricultural Economics* 85(1): 1-15.

Raper, K.C., M.N. Wanzala, and R.M. Nayga. 2002. "Food Expenditures and Household Demographic Composition in the US: A Demand Systems Approach," *Applied Economics* 34(8): 981-992.

Reed, A.J., J.W. Levedahl, and C. Hallahan. 2005. "The Generalized Composite Commodity Theorem and Food Demand Estimation," *American Journal of Agricultural Economics* 87(1): 28-37.

Seale, J.L., M.A. Marchant, and A. Basso. 2003. "Import Versus Domestic Production: A Demand System Analysis of the U.S. Red Wine Market," *Review of Agricultural Economics* 25: 187-202.

Stewart, H., N. Blisard, S. Bhuyan, and R.M. Nayga. 2004. *The Demand for Food Away From Home: Full-Service or Fast Food*? AER-829. U.S. Department of Agriculture, Economic Research Service.

Strotz, R.H. 1957. "The Empirical Implications of a Utility Tree," *Econometrica* 25(2): 269-280.

Strotz, R.H. 1959. "The Utility Tree—A Correction and Further Appraisal," *Econometrica* 27(3): 482-488.

Theil, H. 1965. "The Information Approach to Demand Analysis," *Econometrica* 33(1): 67-87.

Todd, J.E., L. Mancino, and B.-H. Lin. 2010. *The Impact of Food Away From Home on Adult Diet Quality*. ERR-90. U.S. Department of Agriculture, Economic Research Service.

U.S. Department of Agriculture, Economic Research Service. 2011. Food CPI and Expenditures: CPI for Food Forecasts, 2011. http://www.ers.usda.gov/Briefing/CPIFoodAndExpenditures/Data/cpiforecasts.htm.

U.S. Department of Labor, Bureau of Labor Statistics. 2010a. Consumer Expenditure Survey Database. http://data.bls.gov/pdq/querytool.jsp?survey=cx.

U.S. Department of Labor, Bureau of Labor Statistics. 2010b. Consumer Expenditure Survey Public Microdata, 1999-2009: Detailed Expenditure Files.

U.S. Department of Labor, Bureau of Labor Statistics. 2010c. Consumer Price Index

Working, H. 1943. "Statistical Laws of Family Expenditure," *Journal of the American Statistical Association* 38(221): 43-56.

APPENDIX TABLES

Appendix Table A.1. Test for seasonal unit roots in monthly logarithmic transformation of price series

			Seasonal frequency (Tests of coefficients in HEGY test regression)					
	Lag	0 $\pi_1=0$	π $\pi_2=0$	$\pi/2$ $\pi_3=\pi_4=0$	$2\pi/3$ $\pi_5=\pi_6=0$	$\pi/3$ $\pi_7=\pi_8=0$	$5\pi/6$ $\pi 9=\pi 10=^0$	$\pi/6$ $\pi 11=\pi 12=^0$
Cereals and bakery	4	0.02	-2.65	8.53	7.95	9.47	5.04	10.01
Flour and flour mixes	0	-2.29	-2.97	11.00	13.36	14.47	11.56	15.34
Breakfast cereals	2	-1.16	-3.35	11.48	16.92	10.30	8.45	12.44
Rice and pasta	2	0.09	-3.26	8.25	10.55	10.03	7.58	15.71
Nonwhite bread	9	-2.47	-3.71	8.56	9.97	24.58	8.24	10.15
White bread	1	-3.21	-2.40	7.74	9.15	9.35	9.74	12.75
Biscuits, rolls, muffins	1	-2.25	-2.83	8.02	6.41	8.44	10.72	12.01
Cakes and cookies	9	-0.27	-2.05	9.22	10.54	6.09	4.00	11.29
Other bakery products	9	-4.22	-4.53	3.00	11.86	12.48	2.36	7.37
Meat and eggs	0	-2.90	-4.01	9.89	10.24	14.04	11.71	15.58
Beef	0	-1.78	-3.03	11.84	15.86	10.64	11.51	13.57
Pork	13	0.25	-4.73	2.18	1.88	16.39	17.95	7.60
Other red meat	1	-0.39	-4.03	12.40	9.15	11.68	13.17	6.24
Poultry	0	-3.74	-3.58	13.31	12.36	15.08	11.02	11.42
Fish	2	-3.80	-2.69	11.57	10.39	6.20	11.34	12.46
Eggs	3	-0.95	-3.25	9.53	6.41	7.47	5.75	9.09
Dairy	2	-3.45	-3.58	11.15	11.96	11.09	11.44	10.94
Cheese	4	-2.01	-2.41	13.71	8.40	6.43	11.22	4.91
Ice cream	6	-1.41	-2.84	3.67	8.82	8.10	10.20	10.00
Milk	0	-2.96	-3.81	11.39	17.07	14.23	13.66	16.79
Other dairy	2	-2.83	-2.62	13.24	17.77	15.54	9.62	13.85
Fruits and vegetables	6	-0.44	-4.51	4.99	5.88	2.25	9.35	4.42

Appendix Table A.1. (Continued)

			Seasonal frequency (Tests of coefficients in HEGY test regression)					
	Lag	0 $\pi_1=0$	π $\pi_2=0$	$\pi/2$ $\pi_3=\pi_4=0$	$2\pi/3$ $\pi_5=\pi_6=0$	$\pi/3$ $\pi_7=\pi_8=0$	$5\pi/6$ $\pi 9=\pi 10=^0$	$\pi/6$ $\pi 11=\pi 12=^0$
Apples	4	-3.09	-3.21	14.39	9.51	9.72	9.33	11.70
Bananas	11	-1.01	-1.73	9.09	7.85	4.83	9.42	9.56
Citrus	9	-3.43	-1.14	7.35	6.85	2.53	13.18	9.54
Other fresh fruit	11	1.79	-4.73	13.94	13.13	7.55	6.99	6.13
Potatoes	2	-2.92	-2.22	12.67	13.27	11.36	7.68	9.86
Lettuce	16	-3.04	-2.62	18.27	4.74	5.88	27.88	11.35
Tomatoes	3	-2.28	-4.13	8.17	7.95	8.25	7.49	6.78
Other fresh vegetables	1	-0.93	-3.73	10.63	11.30	8.56	8.46	8.16
Proc. fruits & vegetables	1	-2.67	-2.40	6.40	8.07	11.16	12.39	13.92
Nonalcoholic beverages	2	-2.24	-2.64	8.23	10.71	9.65	9.96	12.60
Frozen noncarb. drinks	14	-1.14	-1.58	12.34	7.57	0.54	2.18	2.50
Nonfro noncarb. drinks	4	-4.27	-3.94	20.96	25.76	24.76	26.48	16.64
Carbonated drinks	5	-2.97	-3.69	9.69	16.58	11.72	15.90	20.27
Coffee and tea	9	-3.20	-4.46	8.45	14.32	10.49	2.61	8.73
Sugar and sweets	6	-3.01	-4.33	4.70	3.10	6.18	16.72	4.44
Fats and oils	10	-0.18	-2.82	13.96	7.25	9.36	7.68	4.58
Miscellaneous foods	4	1.72	-3.52	7.66	13.71	8.45	8.99	9.21
Soups	4	-3.44	-3.81	13.07	12.57	17.02	9.07	12.30
Frozen foods	7	-2.53	-3.18	9.42	9.01	8.34	12.96	13.74
Snacks	3	0.03	-2.95	22.36	12.73	11.22	10.66	7.80
Cond., sauces, seas.	2	-2.17	-4.23	4.30	6.54	4.63	13.02	3.59
Other miscellaneous	5	-3.20	-3.09	13.26	8.87	12.24	17.81	7.91
Other FAFH	4	-3.83	-4.53	14.75	17.73	19.15	18.28	26.08
Limited-service FAFH	5	-1.62	-3.44	7.23	7.50	10.40	5.77	8.67

			Seasonal frequency					
			(Tests of coefficients in HEGY test regression)					
		0	π	$\pi/2$	$2\pi/3$	$\pi/3$	$5\pi/6$	$\pi/6$
	Lag	$\pi_1=0$	$\pi_2=0$	$\pi_3=\pi_4=0$	$\pi_5=\pi_6=0$	$\pi_7=\pi_8=0$	$\pi 9=\pi 10=^0$	$\pi 11=\pi 12=^0$
Full-service FAFH	6	-3.50	-3.29	12.70	13.89	8.21	16.55	7.78
Alcoholic beverages	25	-1.04	-4.83	6.44	2.82	1.16	4.38	0.92
Nonfood	4	-2.13	-3.28	10.61	9.89	11.83	11.44	6.13

Note: The HEGY test regressions included a trend, constant, and lagged dependent variables. Beaulieu and Miron (1993) derived the critical values from the distributions of the HEGY test statistics for monthly data. The critical values for the test regression with a trend and a constant and 240 observations for a 10-percent level of significance are:

-2.99 for the test of the null hypothesis $\pi_1 = 0$ versus the alternative $\pi_1 < 0$ (test of long-run unit root), -2.47 for the test of the null hypothesis $\pi_2 = 0$ versus the alternative $\pi_2 < 0$ (test of unit root corresponding to a biannual cycle), and 5.25 for the joint test of the null hypothesis $\pi_n = \pi_{n-1} = 0$, n = 2, 6, 8, 10, 12 (test of unit root corresponding to seasonal frequencies $\pi/2$, $2\pi/3$, $\pi/3$, $5\pi/6$ and $\pi/6$).

FAFH = Food away from home.

Source: Authors' calculation of HEGY test for monthly data using logarithmic transformation of consumer price indexes (U.S. Department of Labor, BLS, Consumer Expenditure Survey (2010a); U.S. Department of Labor, BLS, Consumer Price Index Database (2010c)).

Appendix Table A.2. Test for seasonal unit roots in monthly expenditure share series

			Seasonal frequency					
			(Tests of coefficients in HEGY test regression)					
		0	π	$\pi/2$	$2\pi/3$	$\pi/3$	$5\pi/6$	$\pi/6$
	Lag	$\pi_1=0$	$\pi_2=0$	$\pi_3=\pi_4=0$	$\pi_5=\pi_6=0$	$\pi_7=\pi_8=0$	$\pi 9=\pi 10=^0$	$\pi 11=\pi 12=^0$
Cereals and bakery	6	-1.18	-1.69	12.24	6.72	3.73	12.05	8.98
Flour and flour mixes	3	0.93	-0.46	1.73	0.51	1.73	0.77	3.06
Breakfast cereals	7	-1.28	-3.01	0.89	4.37	1.58	4.47	1.20
Rice and pasta	8	-3.09	-3.61	1.21	9.57	2.30	9.15	2.06
Nonwhite bread	15	-0.10	-0.56	0.90	1.46	15.48	2.44	1.88

Appendix Table A.2. (Continued)

			Seasonal frequency (Tests of coefficients in HEGY test regression)					
	Lag	0 $\pi_1=0$	π $\pi_2=0$	$\pi/2$ $\pi_3=\pi_4=0$	$2\pi/3$ $\pi_5=\pi_6=0$	$\pi/3$ $\pi_7=\pi_8=0$	$5\pi/6$ $\pi 9=\pi 10=^0$	$\pi/6$ $\pi 11=\pi 12=^0$
White bread	1	-0.38	-1.89	8.31	4.81	8.43	11.01	5.11
Biscuits, rolls, muffins	3	-1.49	-1.58	13.80	3.34	5.82	2.57	3.68
Cakes and cookies	6	-3.99	-4.54	14.01	5.09	1.49	10.63	2.65
Other bakery products	17	-2.39	-2.38	0.41	1.69	0.06	0.78	0.28
Meat and eggs	3	-2.90	-4.08	14.16	12.22	9.98	8.24	10.49
Beef	8	-1.86	-1.57	1.57	4.72	4.50	7.03	2.11
Pork	3	-2.32	-1.92	1.85	1.38	5.49	3.55	0.85
Other red meat	3	-1.61	-2.42	9.23	16.00	3.01	13.89	2.05
Poultry	11	-0.53	0.15	0.20	0.98	0.18	0.26	0.05
Fish	4	-2.64	-3.05	11.29	4.07	4.92	6.18	3.17
Eggs	2	-0.77	-3.08	7.97	10.58	10.26	9.18	2.82
Dairy	3	-1.98	-2.58	4.65	7.84	7.88	5.58	2.67
Cheese	9	-4.81	-1.34	2.33	5.59	3.61	1.50	0.02
Ice cream	7	-2.98	-2.70	6.71	7.67	4.10	17.46	0.35
Milk	13	-4.37	-3.31	8.01	1.41	2.83	11.63	0.91
Other dairy	2	-4.11	-4.39	10.89	7.16	6.56	10.28	8.06
Fruits and vegetables	1	-0.45	-2.01	14.98	8.27	4.12	19.85	5.78
Apples	11	-4.02	-1.56	1.90	4.21	0.58	8.55	0.51
Bananas	2	1.83	-1.29	2.28	5.03	2.26	3.02	0.78
Citrus	4	2.42	-1.37	3.57	0.42	1.53	2.88	2.97
Other fresh fruit	4	1.15	-2.33	1.43	1.78	0.67	6.82	0.86
Potatoes	0	-1.81	-3.65	10.34	10.50	5.02	9.07	2.36
Lettuce	9	-1.51	-0.96	1.36	7.56	0.82	6.24	3.52
Tomatoes	2	-2.41	-3.64	3.57	4.71	4.84	3.14	4.08

			Seasonal frequency					
			(Tests of coefficients in HEGY test regression)					
	Lag	0 $\pi_1=0$	π $\pi_2=0$	$\pi/2$ $\pi_3=\pi_4=0$	$2\pi/3$ $\pi_5=\pi_6=0$	$\pi/3$ $\pi_7=\pi_8=0$	$5\pi/6$ $\pi 9=\pi 10=^0$	$\pi/6$ $\pi 11=\pi 12=^0$
Other fresh vegetables	4	-1.31	-3.12	5.96	6.27	4.60	3.18	2.67
Proc. fruits & vegetables	9	0.09	-0.49	8.39	1.09	0.50	2.88	0.37
Nonalcoholic beverages	1	-2.53	-2.75	12.28	11.49	3.96	8.52	7.36
Frozen noncarb. drinks	5	-0.40	-3.49	8.56	1.86	9.00	8.01	13.40
Nonfro. noncarb. drinks	7	0.53	-3.39	5.19	4.14	1.86	4.08	0.13
Carbonated drinks	4	-2.77	-2.92	10.96	2.36	5.74	5.09	9.65
Coffee and tea	4	0.19	-1.62	6.93	2.72	1.99	6.94	1.07
Sugar and sweets	3	-1.98	-2.78	3.32	5.38	2.52	1.40	1.10
Fats and oils	3	1.06	-2.42	3.47	3.25	3.06	4.77	3.56
Miscellaneous foods	4	1.73	-1.85	2.42	1.72	1.74	1.79	0.57
Soups	2	-0.67	-1.09	2.59	2.57	0.84	1.82	1.12
Frozen foods	3	0.85	-1.45	2.29	3.56	4.60	4.02	2.49
Snacks	1	-0.55	-2.44	8.03	9.12	9.89	9.95	6.60
Condiments, sauces, seasonings	2	-2.03	-1.77	2.48	2.81	1.58	2.91	2.47
Other miscellaneous	6	-2.33	-1.57	3.55	2.01	2.51	9.52	0.59
Other FAFH	1	-1.94	-4.40	9.06	11.84	3.05	14.89	2.63
Limited-service FAFH	8	-1.44	-2.91	3.55	0.90	5.50	10.53	1.52
Full-service FAFH	5	-3.60	-1.11	9.09	7.23	10.53	13.76	1.15
Alcoholic beverages	11	-3.44	-1.21	1.55	5.82	0.43	2.14	0.32
Nonfood	2	-3.46	-3.92	10.41	9.55	4.48	12.57	4.06

Note: See notes to table A.1.

Source: Authors' calculation of HEGY test for monthly data using aggregated average monthly household expenditures (U.S. Department of Labor, BLS, Consumer Expenditure Survey (2010a); U.S. Department of Labor, BLS, Consumer Price Index Database (2010c)).

Appendix Table A.3. Second-stage estimated elasticities of demand for cereals and bakery products based on the GODDS model, 1998-2010

Demand for	With respect to price of								With respect to cereals and bakery expenditure	R^2	Breusch-Godfrey statistic	Constant
	Flour and prepared Flour mixes	Break-fast cereals	Rice and pasta	Non-white bread	White bread	Biscuits, rolls,and muffins	Cakes and cookies	Other bakery				
Flour and prepared mixes	0.07	1.20	0.93	-1.96	-0.37	-0.39	-0.98	-0.33	1.82	0.21	1.27	--0.0022
	(0.60)	(0.62)	(0.52)	(0.45)	(0.49)	(0.60)	(0.95)	(0.70)	(0.21)			(0.0008)
Breakfast cereals	0.33	-1.13	-0.09	-0.10	-0.06	0.09	0.50	-0.22	0.68	0.11	0.29	0.0039
	(0.14)	(0.31)	(0.18)	(0.15)	(0.16)	(0.20)	(0.37)	(0.25)	(0.09)			(0.0016)
Rice and pasta	0.41	-0.34	-0.08	-0.10	-0.36	0.20	-0.43	-0.91	1.62	0.21	9.13	-0.0012
	(0.22)	(0.34)	(0.34)	(0.21)	(0.23)	(0.28)	(0.47)	(0.35)	(0.15)			(0.0013)
Non-white bread	-0.71	-0.17	-0.00	-0.64	0.56	-0.09	0.30	0.04	0.72	0.17	0.73	0.0000
	(0.18)	(0.25)	(0.19)	(0.28)	(0.24)	(0.27)	(0.40)	(0.29)	(0.08)			(0.0008)
White bread	-0.18	-0.23	-0.42	0.77	-1.57	-0.09	0.56	0.01	1.16	0.03	13.89	0.0006
	(0.28)	(0.41)	(0.30)	(0.36)	(0.50)	(0.45)	(0.62)	(0.45)	(0.13)			(0.0009)
Biscuits, rolls, and muffins	-0.14	0.16	0.31	-0.11	-0.05	-0.25	-1.00	0.30	0.77	0.05	0.01	-0.0002
	(0.29)	(0.41)	(0.31)	(0.33)	(0.37)	(0.62)	(0.64)	(0.47)	(0.12)			(0.0011)
Cakes and cookies	-0.21	0.44	-0.20	0.14	0.24	-0.55	-1.27	0.24	1.18	0.07	2.80	-0.0005
	(0.23)	(0.40)	(0.27)	(0.25)	(0.27)	(0.33)	(0.74)	(0.43)	(0.12)			(0.0020)
Other bakery	-0.03	-0.24	-0.38	0.01	0.03	0.13	0.27	-0.63	0.85	na	na	na
	(0.15)	(0.23)	(0.17)	(0.16)	(0.17)	(0.21)	(0.38)	(0.35)	(0.08)			

Notes: Estimated elasticities of demand were computed at the mean of the data. Standard errors were bootstrapped using the residual method. Total expenditure includes expenditures on durable and nondurable goods and services. The R^2 and the Breusch-Godfrey statistic are for the individual equations and Breusch-Godfrey statistic is distributed $\chi^2(1)$, for which the 10% critical value is 2.71.

Source: Authors' calculations using iterated feasible generalized least squares (GLS, Stata version 11) with homogeneity and symmetry constraints imposed.

GODDS = Generalized Ordinary Differential Demand System.

Appendix Table A.4. Second-stage estimated elasticities of demand for meat based on the GODDS model, 1998-2010

	With respect to price of						With respect to meat		Breusch-Godfrey	
Demand for	Beef	Pork	Other meat	Poultry	Fish	Eggs	expenditure	R^2	statistic	Constant
Beef	-0.93 (0.19)	0.15 (0.14)	-0.10 (0.12)	-0.17 (0.11)	-0.23 (0.13)	-0.05 (0.03)	1.34 (0.07)	0.18	3.54	0.0009 (0.0022)
Pork	0.30 (0.20)	-1.40 (0.23)	0.09 (0.17)	0.13 (0.15)	-0.16 (0.17)	-0.03 (0.04)	1.08 (0.07)	0.05	4.61	0.0018 (0.0016)
Other red meat	-0.02 (0.26)	0.23 (0.26)	-1.12 (0.41)	-0.13 (0.27)	0.50 (0.29)	-0.10 (0.06)	0.63 (0.09)	0.13	0.28	-0.0012 (0.0013)
Poultry	-0.11 (0.19)	0.21 (0.17)	-0.11 (0.20)	-0.92 (0.24)	0.15 (0.18)	0.01 (0.04)	0.77 (0.06)	0.10	2.51	0.0013 (0.0013)
Fish	-0.34 (0.25)	-0.19 (0.23)	0.40 (0.26)	0.16 (0.22)	-0.94 (0.31)	-0.02 (0.05)	0.93 (0.10)	0.04	1.34	-0.0019 (0.0017)
Eggs	-0.14 (0.19)	-0.07 (0.17)	-0.27 (0.16)	0.05 (0.15)	-0.02 (0.16)	-0.26 (0.06)	0.72 (0.08)	na	na	na

Notes: Estimated elasticities of demand were computed at the mean of the data. Standard errors were bootstrapped using the residual method. Total expenditure includes expenditures on durable and nondurable goods and services. The R^2 and the Breusch-Godfrey statistic are for the individual equations and Breusch-Godfrey statistic is distributed $\chi^2(1)$, for which the 10% critical value is 2.71.

Source: Authors' calculations using iterated feasible generalized least squares (GLS, Stata version 11) with homogeneity and symmetry constraints imposed.

Appendix Table A.5. Second-stage estimated elasticities of demand for dairy based on the GODDS model, 1998-2010

	With respect to price of				With respect		Breusch-	
Demand for	Cheese	Ice cream and frozen desserts	Milk	Other dairy	to dairy expenditure	R^2	Godfrey statistic	Constant
Cheese	-1.02	-0.14	-0.31	0.26	1.21	0.08	1.73	-0.0017
	(0.21)	(0.12)	(0.10)	(0.17)	(0.08)			(0.0017)
Ice cream and related products	-0.25	-0.43	-0.53	0.04	1.18	0.23	0.00	0.0027
	(0.22)	(0.23)	(0.14)	(0.27)	(0.13)			(0.0014)
Milk	-0.14	-0.18	-0.32	-0.15	0.79	0.38	8.79	0.0028
	(0.09)	(0.06)	(0.08)	(0.08)	(0.07)			(0.0016)
Other dairy	0.69	0.10	-0.40	-1.25	0.85	na	na	na
	(0.37)	(0.32)	(0.21)	(0.52)	(0.17)			

Notes: Estimated elasticities of demand were computed at the mean of the data. Standard errors were bootstrapped using the residual method. Total expenditure includes expenditures on durable and nondurable goods and services. The R^2 and the Breusch-Godfrey statistic are for the individual equations and Breusch-Godfrey statistic is distributed $\chi^2(1)$, for which the 10% critical value is 2.71.

Source: Authors' calculations using iterated feasible generalized least squares (GLS, Stata version 11) with homogeneity and symmetry constraints imposed.

Appendix Table A.6. Second-stage estimated elasticities of demand for fruits and vegetables based on the GODDS model, 1998-2010

	With respect to price of									With respect to fruit/veg. expenditure			
Demand for	Apples	Bananas	Citrus	Other fruits	Potatoes	Lettuce	Tomatoes	Other veg.	Processed fruits/ vegetables		R^2	Breusch-Godfrey statistic	Constant
Apples	-0.60	-0.03	0.02	-0.11	-0.11	0.03	-0.05	0.21	-0.13	0.77	0.06	0.01	0.0008
	(0.14)	(0.11)	(0.08)	(0.15)	(0.10)	(0.06)	(0.07)	(0.16)	(0.20)	(0.12)			(0.0007)
Bananas	-0.07	-1.01	-0.11	0.06	0.01	-0.14	-0.05	0.12	-0.05	1.24	0.05	3.04	0.0004
	(0.11)	(0.19)	(0.08)	(0.15)	(0.11)	(0.06)	(0.07)	(0.17)	(0.25)	(0.11)			(0.0006)
Citrus	-0.03	-0.10	-1.09	-0.15	-0.10	0.00	0.10	0.05	-0.09	1.41	0.17	0.98	-0.0008
	(0.07)	(0.07)	(0.09)	(0.13)	(0.07)	(0.04)	(0.06)	(0.12)	(0.15)	(0.12)			(0.0007)
Other fruits	-0.06	0.04	-0.04	-0.93	0.03	-0.05	-0.09	-0.11	0.17	1.03	0.00	34.64	-0.0006
	(0.06)	(0.06)	(0.06)	(0.14)	(0.06)	(0.04)	(0.05)	(0.10)	(0.13)	(0.10)			(0.0014)
Potatoes	-0.11	0.04	-0.07	0.14	-0.45	-0.02	0.10	-0.35	-0.03	0.75	0.17	1.38	0.0007
	(0.11)	(0.11)	(0.08)	(0.15)	(0.14)	(0.06)	(0.07)	(0.16)	(0.21)	(0.12)			(0.0007)
Lettuce	0.02	-0.17	0.03	-0.16	-0.04	-0.85	0.05	0.12	-0.01	1.01	0.05	1.41	-0.0001
	(0.08)	(0.08)	(0.07)	(0.13)	(0.08)	(0.07)	(0.06)	(0.13)	(0.16)	(0.10)			(0.0004)
Tomatoes	-0.10	-0.06	0.11	-0.29	0.05	0.01	-0.57	0.00	-0.58	1.43	0.28	1.34	0.0002
	(0.07)	(0.07)	(0.06)	(0.12)	(0.07)	(0.04)	(0.08)	(0.12)	(0.15)	(0.12)			(0.0007)
Other vegetables	0.06	0.05	0.05	-0.09	-0.14	0.03	0.03	-0.98	-0.03	1.01	0.02	6.88	0.0010
	(0.06)	(0.06)	(0.05)	(0.09)	(0.05)	(0.03)	(0.04)	(0.12)	(0.12)	(0.08)			(0.0012)
Processed fruits/ vegetables	-0.04	0.02	0.02	0.18	-0.01	0.01	-0.13	0.03	-0.84	0.77	na	na	na
	(0.06)	(0.07)	(0.05)	(0.09)	(0.06)	(0.03)	(0.04)	(0.09)	(0.16)	(0.09)			

Notes: Estimated elasticities of demand were computed at the mean of the data. Standard errors were bootstrapped using the residual method. Total expenditure includes expenditures on durable and nondurable goods and services. The R^2 and the Breusch-Godfrey statistic are for the individual equations and Breusch-Godfrey statistic is distributed $\chi^2(1)$, for which the 10% critical value is 2.71.

Source: Authors' calculations using iterated feasible generalized least squares (GLS, Stata version 11) with homogeneity and symmetry constraints imposed.

Appendix Table A.7. Second-stage estimated elasticities of demand for nonalcoholic beverages based on the GODDS (Generalized Ordinary Differential Demand System) model, 1998-2010

	With respect to price of						
Demand for	Coffee and tea	Carbonated beverages	Nonfrozen noncarbon- ated juices and drinks	Frozen non-carbonated juices and drinks	With respect to nonalcoholic beverage expenditure	R^2	Constant
Coffee and tea	-0.17 (0.26)	-0.07 (0.31)	-0.31 (0.30)	-0.01 (0.08)	0.56 (0.14)	0.25	-0.0042 (0.0017)
Carbonated beverages	-0.12 (0.15)	-0.58 (0.34)	-0.37 (0.30)	0.01 (0.07)	1.06 (0.09)	0.01	0.0074 (0.0024)
Nonfrozen noncarbonated juices and drinks	-0.22 (0.11)	-0.31 (0.23)	-0.61 (0.27)	0.01 (0.07)	1.13 (0.07)	0.18	-0.0048 (0.0024)
Frozen noncarbonated juices and drinks	-0.14 (0.59)	0.25 (1.11)	0.38 (1.36)	-1.37 (0.91)	0.88 (0.33)	na	na

Notes: Estimated elasticities of demand were computed at the mean of the data. Standard errors were bootstrapped using the residual method. Total expenditure includes expenditures on durable and nondurable goods and services. The R^2 values are for the individual equations. Source: Authors' calculations using iterated feasible generalized least squares (GLS, Stata version 11) with homogeneity and symmetry constraints imposed and with correction for first-order autocorrelation.

Appendix Table A.8. Second-stage estimated elasticities of demand for other FAH based on the GODDS model, 1998-2010

Demand for	With respect to price of: Sugar and sweets	Fats and oils	Soups	Frozen foods	Snacks	Condiments, sauces, seasonings	Miscel-laneous	With respect to other FAH expenditure	R^2	Breusch-Godfrey statistic	Constant
Sugar and sweets	-0.47	-0.06	-0.70	-0.75	0.02	0.63	-0.06	1.39	0.08	0.41	0.0086
	(0.73)	(0.23)	(0.23)	(0.46)	(0.14)	(0.35)	(0.56)	(0.18)			(0.0028)
Fats and oils	0.04	-0.24	-0.19	-0.24	0.02	0.06	-0.27	0.83	0.19	2.06	0.0037
	(0.25)	(0.16)	(0.10)	(0.22)	(0.06)	(0.14)	(0.25)	(0.10)			(0.0013)
Soups	-2.05	-0.48	0.18	0.96	0.05	0.30	0.59	0.45	0.04	0.01	-0.0018
	(0.72)	(0.28)	(0.56)	(0.68)	(0.27)	(0.58)	(0.67)	(0.18)			(0.0009)
Frozen foods	-0.74	-0.26	0.30	-1.06	-0.23	0.07	0.95	0.96	0.05	0.75	-0.0038
	(0.50)	(0.22)	(0.24)	(0.62)	(0.14)	(0.35)	(0.47)	(0.14)			(0.0021)
Snacks	0.22	0.11	0.07	-1.01	-1.15	1.06	-0.10	0.81	0.04	1.31	0.0000
	(0.70)	(0.27)	(0.42)	(0.65)	(0.47)	(0.60)	(0.60)	(0.16)			(0.0005)
Condiments, sauces, seasonings	0.89	0.08	0.10	0.12	0.26	-1.95	-0.25	0.75	0.12	0.80	0.0008
	(0.42)	(0.16)	(0.22)	(0.39)	(0.15)	(0.44)	(0.37)	(0.10)			(0.0013)
Miscellaneous	-0.01	-0.27	0.11	0.69	-0.03	-0.24	-1.44	1.18	na	na	na
	(0.46)	(0.18)	(0.18)	(0.36)	(0.10)	(0.25)	(0.55)	(0.14)			

Notes: Estimated elasticities of demand were computed at the mean of the data. Standard errors were bootstrapped using the residual method. Total expenditure includes expenditures on durable and nondurable goods and services. The R^2 and the Breusch-Godfrey statistic are for the individual equations and Breusch-Godfrey statistic is distributed $\chi^2(1)$, for which the 10% critical value is 2.71.

Source: Authors' calculations using iterated feasible GLS (Stata version 11) with homogeneity and symmetry constraints imposed.

Appendix Table A.9. Second-stage estimated elasticities of demand for FAFH (food away from home) and alcohol based on the GODDS model, 1998-2010

	With respect to price of				With respect to FAFH and alcohol expenditure			
Demand for	Alcohol	Limited-service	Full-service	Other FAFH		R^2	Breusch-Godfrey statistic	Constant
Alcohol	-1.13 (0.63)	-2.39 (0.66)	2.17 (0.74)	-0.16 (0.12)	1.53 (0.16)	0.10	6.24	-0.0021 (0.0020)
Limited-service	-0.89 (0.27)	-0.26 (0.94)	0.31 (0.95)	-0.00 (0.06)	0.84 (0.07)	0.15	4.25	0.0057 (0.0024)
Full-service	0.92 (0.29)	0.24 (0.88)	-2.08 (0.96)	-0.02 (0.06)	0.94 (0.08)	0.08	21.87	-0.0054 (0.0027)
Other FAFH	-0.31 (0.37)	-0.06 (0.32)	-0.17 (0.21)	-0.45 (0.52)	0.98 (0.17)	na	na	na

Notes: Estimated elasticities of demand were computed at the mean of the data. Standard errors were bootstrapped using the residual method. Total expenditure includes expenditures on durable and nondurable goods and services. The R^2 and the Breusch-Godfrey statistic are for the individual equations and Breusch-Godfrey statistic is distributed $\chi^2(1)$, for which the 10% critical value is 2.71.

Source: Authors' calculations using iterated feasible GLS (Stata version 11) with homogeneity and symmetry constraints imposed.

FAFH = Food away from home, including limited-service and full-service restaurants; FAH = Food at home; GODDS = Generalized Ordinary Differential Demand System.

Appendix Table A.10. Estimated unconditional elasticities of demand

	With respect to price of							
Demand for	Flour, prep. mixes	Breakfast cereals	Rice and pasta	Nonwhite bread	White bread	Biscuits, rolls, muff.	Cakes and cookies	Other bakery products
Flour, prep. mixes	0.07	1.41	0.94	-1.84	-0.32	-0.30	-0.88	-0.14
	(0.71)	(0.67)	(0.56)	(0.51)	(0.58)	(0.68)	(1.09)	(0.74)
Breakfast cereals	0.32	-1.05	-0.08	-0.05	-0.04	0.12	0.54	-0.15
	(0.15)	(0.33)	(0.19)	(0.17)	(0.18)	(0.21)	(0.40)	(0.25)
Rice and pasta	0.41	-0.15	-0.07	0.00	-0.31	0.28	-0.34	-0.75
	(0.24)	(0.36)	(0.38)	(0.22)	(0.27)	(0.30)	(0.53)	(0.36)
Nonwhite bread	-0.72	-0.09	0.00	-0.59	0.58	-0.05	0.34	0.11
	(0.20)	(0.28)	(0.20)	(0.30)	(0.28)	(0.31)	(0.45)	(0.31)
White bread	-0.18	-0.10	-0.42	0.84	-1.54	-0.04	0.63	0.13
	(0.33)	(0.44)	(0.35)	(0.41)	(0.58)	(0.54)	(0.69)	(0.47)
Biscuits, rolls, muff.	-0.14	0.25	0.31	-0.06	-0.03	-0.21	-0.95	0.38
	(0.33)	(0.44)	(0.34)	(0.38)	(0.45)	(0.71)	(0.72)	(0.47)
Cakes and cookies	-0.22	0.57	-0.19	0.21	0.27	-0.49	-1.20	0.36
	(0.27)	(0.43)	(0.30)	(0.28)	(0.30)	(0.37)	(0.81)	(0.42)
Other bakery	-0.03	-0.14	-0.37	0.06	0.05	0.17	0.31	-0.55
	(0.16)	(0.23)	(0.18)	(0.17)	(0.18)	(0.21)	(0.37)	(0.34)
Beef	0.00	0.01	0.01	0.00	0.00	0.00	0.01	0.01
	(0.01)	(0.01)	(0.02)	(0.01)	(0.01)	(0.01)	(0.02)	(0.02)
Pork	0.00	0.00	0.01	0.00	0.00	0.00	0.01	0.01
	(0.01)	(0.01)	(0.01)	(0.01)	(0.01)	(0.01)	(0.02)	(0.01)
Other red meat	0.00	0.00	0.00	0.00	0.00	0.00	0.00	0.00
	(0.00)	(0.01)	(0.01)	(0.00)	(0.00)	(0.00)	(0.01)	(0.01)
Poultry	0.00	0.00	0.00	0.00	0.00	0.00	0.00	0.00
	(0.00)	(0.01)	(0.01)	(0.00)	(0.01)	(0.00)	(0.01)	(0.01)
Fish	0.00	0.00	0.00	0.00	0.00	0.00	0.01	0.00
	(0.01)	(0.01)	(0.01)	(0.01)	(0.01)	(0.00)	(0.01)	(0.01)

See notes at end of table.

Appendix Table A.10. (Continued)

	With respect to price of								
Demand for	Beef	Pork	Other red meat	Poultry	Fish	Eggs	Cheese	Ice cream and frozen desserts	Milk
Flour, prep. mixes	0.04	0.02	0.01	0.01	0.01	0.00	0.24	0.13	0.19
	(0.09)	(0.05)	(0.02)	(0.03)	(0.03)	(0.01)	(0.07)	(0.04)	(0.06)
Breakfast cereals	0.01	0.01	0.00	0.01	0.00	0.00	0.09	0.05	0.07
	(0.03)	(0.02)	(0.01)	(0.01)	(0.01)	(0.00)	(0.03)	(0.01)	(0.02)
Rice and pasta	0.03	0.02	0.01	0.01	0.01	0.00	0.22	0.12	0.17
	(0.08)	(0.04)	(0.02)	(0.03)	(0.03)	(0.01)	(0.06)	(0.03)	(0.05)
Nonwhite bread	0.01	0.01	0.00	0.01	0.01	0.00	0.10	0.05	0.08
	(0.04)	(0.02)	(0.01)	(0.01)	(0.01)	(0.00)	(0.03)	(0.01)	(0.02)
White bread	0.02	0.01	0.01	0.01	0.01	0.00	0.15	0.08	0.12
	(0.06)	(0.03)	(0.01)	(0.02)	(0.02)	(0.01)	(0.05)	(0.03)	(0.03)
Biscuits, rolls, muff.	0.02	0.01	0.00	0.01	0.01	0.00	0.10	0.06	0.08
	(0.04)	(0.02)	(0.01)	(0.01)	(0.01)	(0.00)	(0.03)	(0.02)	(0.02)
Cakes and cookies	0.02	0.01	0.01	0.01	0.01	0.00	0.16	0.08	0.12
	(0.06)	(0.03)	(0.01)	(0.02)	(0.02)	(0.01)	(0.05)	(0.03)	(0.04)
Other bakery	0.02	0.01	0.00	0.01	0.01	0.00	0.11	0.06	0.09
	(0.04)	(0.02)	(0.01)	(0.02)	(0.02)	(0.00)	(0.03)	(0.02)	(0.02)
Beef	-0.70	0.33	0.04	0.01	-0.09	0.00	0.01	0.01	0.01
	(0.20)	(0.15)	(0.11)	(0.12)	(0.12)	(0.03)	(0.03)	(0.01)	(0.02)
Pork	0.48	-1.26	0.20	0.28	-0.05	0.01	0.01	0.01	0.01
	(0.21)	(0.26)	(0.18)	(0.18)	(0.17)	(0.04)	(0.02)	(0.01)	(0.02)
Other red meat	0.09	0.32	-1.05	-0.04	0.56	-0.07	0.01	0.00	0.00
	(0.26)	(0.28)	(0.42)	(0.30)	(0.29)	(0.07)	(0.01)	(0.01)	(0.01)
Poultry	0.02	0.31	-0.03	-0.81	0.23	0.04	0.01	0.00	0.01
	(0.19)	(0.20)	(0.22)	(0.28)	(0.19)	(0.04)	(0.02)	(0.01)	(0.01)
Fish	-0.18	-0.06	0.50	0.28	-0.84	0.02	0.01	0.00	0.01
	(0.24)	(0.24)	(0.25)	(0.23)	(0.30)	(0.06)	(0.02)	(0.01)	(0.01)

	With respect to price of								
Demand for	Other dairy	Apples	Bananas	Citrus	Other fresh fruits	Potatoes	Lettuce	Tomatoes	Other fresh vegetable
Flour, prep. mixes	0.08	-0.03	-0.05	-0.06	-0.10	-0.03	-0.03	-0.06	-0.11
	(0.03)	(0.01)	(0.02)	(0.03)	(0.05)	(0.01)	(0.01)	(0.03)	(0.05)
Breakfast cereals	0.03	-0.01	-0.02	-0.02	-0.04	-0.01	-0.01	-0.02	-0.04
	(0.01)	(0.01)	(0.01)	(0.01)	(0.02)	(0.01)	(0.01)	(0.01)	(0.02)
Rice and pasta	0.07	-0.03	-0.04	-0.06	-0.09	-0.03	-0.02	-0.05	-0.10
	(0.02)	(0.01)	(0.02)	(0.03)	(0.04)	(0.01)	(0.01)	(0.02)	(0.05)
Nonwhite bread	0.03	-0.01	-0.02	-0.02	-0.04	-0.01	-0.01	-0.02	-0.04
	(0.01)	(0.01)	(0.01)	(0.01)	(0.02)	(0.01)	(0.01)	(0.01)	(0.02)
White bread	0.05	-0.02	-0.03	-0.04	-0.06	-0.02	-0.02	-0.04	-0.07
	(0.02)	(0.01)	(0.01)	(0.02)	(0.03)	(0.01)	(0.01)	(0.02)	(0.03)
Biscuits, rolls, muff.	0.04	-0.01	-0.02	-0.03	-0.04	-0.01	-0.01	-0.02	-0.05
	(0.01)	(0.01)	(0.01)	(0.01)	(0.02)	(0.01)	(0.01)	(0.01)	(0.02)
Cakes and cookies	0.05	-0.02	-0.03	-0.04	-0.07	-0.02	-0.02	-0.04	-0.07
	(0.02)	(0.01)	(0.01)	(0.02)	(0.03)	(0.01)	(0.01)	(0.02)	(0.03)
Other bakery	0.04	-0.01	-0.02	-0.03	-0.05	-0.01	-0.01	-0.03	-0.05
	(0.01)	(0.01)	(0.01)	(0.01)	(0.02)	(0.01)	(0.01)	(0.01)	(0.02)
Beef	0.00	0.01	0.01	0.02	0.03	0.01	0.01	0.01	0.03
	(0.01)	(0.01)	(0.01)	(0.01)	(0.02)	(0.01)	(0.01)	(0.01)	(0.03)
Pork	0.00	0.01	0.01	0.01	0.02	0.01	0.01	0.01	0.02
	(0.01)	(0.01)	(0.01)	(0.01)	(0.02)	(0.01)	(0.01)	(0.01)	(0.02)
Other red meat	0.00	0.00	0.01	0.01	0.01	0.00	0.00	0.01	0.01
	(0.00)	(0.00)	(0.00)	(0.01)	(0.01)	(0.00)	(0.00)	(0.01)	(0.01)
Poultry	0.00	0.00	0.01	0.01	0.02	0.00	0.00	0.01	0.02
	(0.01)	(0.00)	(0.01)	(0.01)	(0.01)	(0.00)	(0.00)	(0.01)	(0.01)
Fish	0.00	0.01	0.01	0.01	0.02	0.01	0.00	0.01	0.02
	(0.01)	(0.00)	(0.01)	(0.01)	(0.02)	(0.00)	(0.00)	(0.01)	(0.02)

Appendix Table A.10. (Continued)

				With respect to price of					
Demand for	Processed fruits and vegetables	Coffee and tea	Carbonated beverages	Non-carbonated beverages	Frozen beverages	Sugar and sweets	Fats and oils	Soups	Snacks
Flour, prep.	-0.10	-0.02	-0.06	-0.09	0.00	0.12	0.06	0.01	0.01
mixes	(0.05)	(0.03)	(0.12)	(0.17)	(0.01)	(0.16)	(0.09)	(0.02)	(0.02)
Breakfast	-0.04	-0.01	-0.02	-0.03	0.00	0.04	0.02	0.00	0.01
cereals	(0.02)	(0.01)	(0.04)	(0.06)	(0.00)	(0.06)	(0.03)	(0.01)	(0.01)
Rice and pasta	-0.09	-0.02	-0.06	-0.08	0.00	0.10	0.06	0.01	0.01
	(0.04)	(0.03)	(0.11)	(0.15)	(0.01)	(0.15)	(0.08)	(0.02)	(0.02)
Nonwhite	-0.04	-0.01	-0.03	-0.03	0.00	0.05	0.02	0.00	0.01
bread	(0.02)	(0.01)	(0.05)	(0.07)	(0.00)	(0.06)	(0.03)	(0.01)	(0.01)
White bread	-0.06	-0.01	-0.04	-0.06	0.00	0.07	0.04	0.01	0.01
	(0.03)	(0.02)	(0.08)	(0.11)	(0.00)	(0.10)	(0.06)	(0.01)	(0.01)
Biscuits, rolls,	-0.04	-0.01	-0.03	-0.04	0.00	0.05	0.03	0.01	0.01
muff.	(0.02)	(0.01)	(0.05)	(0.07)	(0.00)	(0.07)	(0.04)	(0.01)	(0.01)
Cakes and	-0.07	-0.01	-0.04	-0.06	0.00	0.08	0.04	0.01	0.01
cookies	(0.03)	(0.02)	(0.08)	(0.11)	(0.00)	(0.11)	(0.06)	(0.01)	(0.01)
Other bakery	-0.05	-0.01	-0.03	-0.04	0.00	0.05	0.03	0.01	0.01
	(0.02)	(0.01)	(0.06)	(0.08)	(0.00)	(0.08)	(0.04)	(0.01)	(0.01)
Beef	0.03	0.01	0.04	0.05	0.00	0.09	0.05	0.01	0.01
	(0.02)	(0.01)	(0.02)	(0.03)	(0.00)	(0.04)	(0.02)	(0.01)	(0.01)
Pork	0.02	0.01	0.03	0.04	0.00	0.07	0.04	0.01	0.01
	(0.02)	(0.00)	(0.02)	(0.03)	(0.00)	(0.03)	(0.02)	(0.00)	(0.00)
Other red meat	0.01	0.00	0.02	0.03	0.00	0.04	0.02	0.00	0.00
	(0.01)	(0.00)	(0.01)	(0.02)	(0.00)	(0.02)	(0.01)	(0.00)	(0.00)
Poultry	0.01	0.01	0.02	0.03	0.00	0.05	0.03	0.01	0.01
	(0.01)	(0.00)	(0.01)	(0.02)	(0.00)	(0.03)	(0.01)	(0.00)	(0.00)
Fish	0.02	0.01	0.03	0.04	0.00	0.06	0.03	0.01	0.01
	(0.02)	(0.00)	(0.02)	(0.02)	(0.00)	(0.03)	(0.02)	(0.00)	(0.00)

	With respect to price of							
Demand for	Condiments, sauces, season.	Miscellaneous FAH	Alcoholic beverages	Limited-service FAFH	Full-service FAFH	Other FAFH	Nonfood	With respect to expenditure
Flour, prep. mixes	0.05	0.12	0.07	0.09	0.11	0.02	0.30	0.01
	(0.07)	(0.16)	(0.17)	(0.22)	(0.27)	(0.05)	(0.61)	(0.08)
Breakfast cereals	0.02	0.04	0.03	0.03	0.04	0.01	0.11	0.00
	(0.03)	(0.06)	(0.06)	(0.08)	(0.10)	(0.02)	(0.23)	(0.03)
Rice and pasta	0.05	0.11	0.06	0.08	0.10	0.02	0.26	0.01
	(0.06)	(0.14)	(0.15)	(0.20)	(0.24)	(0.04)	(0.54)	(0.08)
Nonwhite bread	0.02	0.05	0.03	0.04	0.04	0.01	0.12	0.00
	(0.03)	(0.06)	(0.07)	(0.09)	(0.11)	(0.02)	(0.24)	(0.03)
White bread	0.03	0.08	0.04	0.06	0.07	0.01	0.19	0.01
	(0.05)	(0.10)	(0.11)	(0.14)	(0.17)	(0.03)	(0.39)	(0.05)
Biscuits, rolls, muff.	0.02	0.05	0.03	0.04	0.05	0.01	0.13	0.00
	(0.03)	(0.07)	(0.07)	(0.10)	(0.12)	(0.02)	(0.26)	(0.04)
Cakes and cookies	0.03	0.08	0.04	0.06	0.07	0.01	0.19	0.01
	(0.05)	(0.11)	(0.11)	(0.14)	(0.18)	(0.03)	(0.39)	(0.05)
Other bakery	0.02	0.06	0.03	0.04	0.05	0.01	0.14	0.00
	(0.03)	(0.08)	(0.08)	(0.10)	(0.13)	(0.02)	(0.28)	(0.04)
Beef	0.04	0.09	0.06	0.07	0.09	0.01	-0.54	0.05
	(0.02)	(0.04)	(0.11)	(0.14)	(0.18)	(0.03)	(0.60)	(0.09)
Pork	0.03	0.07	0.04	0.06	0.07	0.01	-0.43	0.04
	(0.02)	(0.03)	(0.09)	(0.11)	(0.14)	(0.02)	(0.48)	(0.07)
Other red meat	0.02	0.04	0.03	0.03	0.04	0.01	-0.25	0.02
	(0.01)	(0.02)	(0.05)	(0.07)	(0.08)	(0.01)	(0.29)	(0.04)
Poultry	0.02	0.05	0.03	0.04	0.05	0.01	-0.31	0.03
	(0.01)	(0.02)	(0.06)	(0.08)	(0.10)	(0.02)	(0.35)	(0.05)
Fish	0.03	0.06	0.04	0.05	0.06	0.01	-0.37	0.03
	(0.01)	(0.03)	(0.08)	(0.10)	(0.12)	(0.02)	(0.42)	(0.06)

Appendix Table A.10. (Continued)

	With respect to price of								
Demand for	Flour, prep. mixes	Breakfast cereals	Rice and pasta	Non-white bread	White bread	Biscuits, rolls, muff.	Cakes and cookies	Other bakery products	Beef
Eggs	0.00	0.00	0.00	0.00	0.00	0.00	0.00	0.00	-0.02
	(0.00)	(0.01)	(0.01)	(0.00)	(0.00)	(0.00)	(0.01)	(0.01)	(0.20)
Cheese	0.05	0.07	0.09	0.05	0.05	0.04	0.12	0.10	0.03
	(0.01)	(0.02)	(0.03)	(0.01)	(0.02)	(0.01)	(0.04)	(0.03)	(0.06)
Ice cream and froz. dessert	0.05	0.07	0.09	0.05	0.05	0.04	0.12	0.10	0.03
	(0.01)	(0.02)	(0.03)	(0.01)	(0.02)	(0.01)	(0.04)	(0.03)	(0.06)
Milk	0.03	0.05	0.06	0.03	0.04	0.03	0.08	0.07	0.02
	(0.01)	(0.01)	(0.02)	(0.01)	(0.01)	(0.01)	(0.02)	(0.02)	(0.04)
Other dairy	0.04	0.06	0.07	0.04	0.04	0.03	0.09	0.08	0.02
	(0.01)	(0.02)	(0.02)	(0.01)	(0.01)	(0.01)	(0.03)	(0.02)	(0.04)
Apples	-0.02	-0.03	-0.04	-0.02	-0.02	-0.02	-0.05	-0.04	0.06
	(0.01)	(0.02)	(0.02)	(0.01)	(0.01)	(0.01)	(0.02)	(0.02)	(0.05)
Bananas	-0.03	-0.05	-0.06	-0.03	-0.03	-0.03	-0.08	-0.07	0.09
	(0.01)	(0.02)	(0.03)	(0.01)	(0.02)	(0.01)	(0.04)	(0.03)	(0.08)
Citrus	-0.03	-0.06	-0.07	-0.03	-0.04	-0.03	-0.09	-0.07	0.10
	(0.02)	(0.03)	(0.03)	(0.02)	(0.02)	(0.02)	(0.04)	(0.04)	(0.09)
Other fresh fruits	-0.03	-0.04	-0.05	-0.03	-0.03	-0.02	-0.07	-0.05	0.07
	(0.01)	(0.02)	(0.02)	(0.01)	(0.01)	(0.01)	(0.03)	(0.03)	(0.07)
Potatoes	-0.02	-0.03	-0.04	-0.02	-0.02	-0.02	-0.05	-0.04	0.05
	(0.01)	(0.01)	(0.02)	(0.01)	(0.01)	(0.01)	(0.02)	(0.02)	(0.05)
Lettuce	-0.02	-0.04	-0.05	-0.02	-0.03	-0.02	-0.06	-0.05	0.07
	(0.01)	(0.02)	(0.03)	(0.01)	(0.01)	(0.01)	(0.03)	(0.03)	(0.06)
Tomatoes	-0.03	-0.06	-0.07	-0.04	-0.04	-0.03	-0.09	-0.08	0.10
	(0.02)	(0.03)	(0.04)	(0.02)	(0.02)	(0.02)	(0.04)	(0.04)	(0.09)
Other fresh vegetables	-0.02	-0.04	-0.05	-0.02	-0.03	-0.02	-0.07	-0.05	0.07
	(0.01)	(0.02)	(0.02)	(0.01)	(0.01)	(0.01)	(0.03)	(0.03)	(0.06)

					With respect to price of					
Demand for	Pork	Other red meat	Poultry	Fish	Eggs	Cheese	Ice cream and frozen desserts	Milk	Other dairy	Apples
Eggs	0.03	-0.20	0.15	0.06	-0.24	0.01	0.00	0.01	0.00	0.00
	(0.19)	(0.18)	(0.17)	(0.17)	(0.06)	(0.01)	(0.01)	(0.01)	(0.00)	(0.00)
Cheese	0.01	0.01	0.01	0.01	0.00	-0.70	0.07	0.15	0.42	0.00
	(0.03)	(0.01)	(0.02)	(0.02)	(0.01)	(0.24)	(0.13)	(0.13)	(0.19)	(0.01)
Ice cream and	0.01	0.01	0.01	0.01	0.00	0.13	-0.23	-0.08	0.12	0.00
froz. dessert	(0.03)	(0.01)	(0.02)	(0.02)	(0.01)	(0.24)	(0.22)	(0.16)	(0.25)	(0.01)
Milk	0.01	0.00	0.01	0.01	0.00	0.13	-0.04	-0.10	-0.03	0.00
	(0.02)	(0.01)	(0.01)	(0.01)	(0.00)	(0.11)	(0.07)	(0.09)	(0.09)	(0.01)
Other dairy	0.01	0.00	0.01	0.01	0.00	0.93	0.14	-0.08	-1.04	0.00
	(0.02)	(0.01)	(0.02)	(0.02)	(0.00)	(0.42)	(0.29)	(0.23)	(0.53)	(0.01)
Apples	0.03	0.01	0.02	0.02	0.00	-0.01	0.00	0.00	0.00	-0.58
	(0.03)	(0.01)	(0.02)	(0.02)	(0.00)	(0.03)	(0.01)	(0.02)	(0.01)	(0.16)
Bananas	0.05	0.02	0.03	0.03	0.01	-0.01	0.00	-0.01	0.00	-0.03
	(0.04)	(0.02)	(0.03)	(0.03)	(0.01)	(0.04)	(0.02)	(0.03)	(0.01)	(0.12)
Citrus	0.06	0.02	0.04	0.04	0.01	-0.01	-0.01	-0.01	0.00	0.01
	(0.05)	(0.02)	(0.03)	(0.03)	(0.01)	(0.05)	(0.03)	(0.04)	(0.02)	(0.09)
Other fresh fruits	0.04	0.02	0.03	0.03	0.01	-0.01	0.00	-0.01	0.00	-0.03
	(0.04)	(0.01)	(0.02)	(0.02)	(0.01)	(0.04)	(0.02)	(0.03)	(0.01)	(0.07)
Potatoes	0.03	0.01	0.02	0.02	0.00	-0.01	0.00	0.00	0.00	-0.09
	(0.03)	(0.01)	(0.02)	(0.02)	(0.00)	(0.03)	(0.01)	(0.02)	(0.01)	(0.11)
Lettuce	0.04	0.02	0.03	0.03	0.01	-0.01	0.00	-0.01	0.00	0.05
	(0.04)	(0.01)	(0.02)	(0.02)	(0.01)	(0.03)	(0.02)	(0.03)	(0.01)	(0.09)
Tomatoes	0.06	0.02	0.04	0.04	0.01	-0.01	-0.01	-0.01	0.00	-0.06
	(0.05)	(0.02)	(0.03)	(0.03)	(0.01)	(0.05)	(0.03)	(0.04)	(0.02)	(0.08)
Other fresh	0.04	0.02	0.03	0.03	0.01	-0.01	0.00	-0.01	0.00	0.09
vegetables	(0.04)	(0.01)	(0.02)	(0.02)	(0.01)	(0.03)	(0.02)	(0.03)	(0.01)	(0.06)

Appendix Table A.10. (Continued)

				With respect to price of					
Demand for	Bananas	Citrus	Other fresh fruits	Potatoes	Lettuce	Tomatoes	Other fresh vegetable	Processed fruits and vegetables	Coffee and tea
Eggs	0.01	0.01	0.01	0.00	0.00	0.01	0.02	0.01	0.01
	(0.01)	(0.01)	(0.01)	(0.00)	(0.00)	(0.01)	(0.01)	(0.01)	(0.00)
Cheese	0.00	0.00	-0.01	0.00	0.00	0.00	-0.01	-0.01	-0.02
	(0.01)	(0.02)	(0.03)	(0.01)	(0.01)	(0.02)	(0.03)	(0.03)	(0.01)
Ice cream and	0.00	0.00	-0.01	0.00	0.00	0.00	-0.01	-0.01	-0.02
froz. dessert	(0.01)	(0.02)	(0.03)	(0.01)	(0.01)	(0.01)	(0.03)	(0.03)	(0.01)
Milk	0.00	0.00	0.00	0.00	0.00	0.00	0.00	0.00	-0.01
	(0.01)	(0.01)	(0.02)	(0.01)	(0.00)	(0.01)	(0.02)	(0.02)	(0.01)
Other dairy	0.00	0.00	0.00	0.00	0.00	0.00	0.00	0.00	-0.01
	(0.01)	(0.01)	(0.02)	(0.01)	(0.01)	(0.01)	(0.02)	(0.02)	(0.01)
Apples	-0.03	0.01	-0.08	-0.09	0.03	-0.06	0.24	-0.06	0.00
	(0.12)	(0.10)	(0.17)	(0.11)	(0.06)	(0.08)	(0.17)	(0.22)	(0.01)
Bananas	-1.01	-0.12	0.10	0.05	-0.13	-0.06	0.16	0.06	0.00
	(0.21)	(0.10)	(0.18)	(0.12)	(0.07)	(0.08)	(0.19)	(0.28)	(0.01)
Citrus	-0.10	-1.10	-0.11	-0.06	0.02	0.09	0.10	0.04	0.00
	(0.08)	(0.10)	(0.15)	(0.08)	(0.05)	(0.07)	(0.13)	(0.17)	(0.01)
Other fresh fruits	0.04	-0.05	-0.90	0.06	-0.04	-0.10	-0.07	0.27	0.00
	(0.07)	(0.07)	(0.15)	(0.07)	(0.04)	(0.06)	(0.11)	(0.14)	(0.01)
Potatoes	0.04	-0.07	0.16	-0.42	-0.01	0.09	-0.32	0.03	0.00
	(0.12)	(0.09)	(0.17)	(0.15)	(0.06)	(0.08)	(0.17)	(0.23)	(0.01)
Lettuce	-0.17	0.03	-0.13	-0.01	-0.84	0.04	0.16	0.08	0.00
	(0.09)	(0.08)	(0.14)	(0.09)	(0.07)	(0.07)	(0.15)	(0.18)	(0.01)
Tomatoes	-0.06	0.10	-0.24	0.09	0.03	-0.58	0.06	-0.45	0.00
	(0.08)	(0.08)	(0.15)	(0.07)	(0.05)	(0.09)	(0.14)	(0.17)	(0.01)
Other fresh	0.06	0.04	-0.06	-0.11	0.04	0.02	-0.94	0.07	0.00
vegetables	(0.06)	(0.05)	(0.10)	(0.06)	(0.04)	(0.05)	(0.14)	(0.13)	(0.01)

Demand for	With respect to price of							
	Carbonated beverages	Non-carbonated beverages	Frozen beverages	Sugar and sweets	Fats and oils	Soups	Frozen meals and snacks	Snacks
Eggs	0.02	0.03	0.00	0.05	0.03	0.00	0.03	0.01
	(0.01)	(0.02)	(0.00)	(0.02)	(0.01)	(0.00)	(0.01)	(0.00)
Cheese	-0.07	-0.09	0.00	-0.13	-0.07	-0.01	-0.08	-0.02
	(0.04)	(0.05)	(0.00)	(0.06)	(0.03)	(0.01)	(0.04)	(0.01)
Ice cream and froz. dessert	-0.07	-0.09	0.00	-0.13	-0.07	-0.01	-0.08	-0.02
	(0.04)	(0.05)	(0.00)	(0.06)	(0.03)	(0.01)	(0.04)	(0.01)
Milk	-0.05	-0.06	0.00	-0.09	-0.05	-0.01	-0.06	-0.01
	(0.02)	(0.04)	(0.00)	(0.04)	(0.02)	(0.01)	(0.03)	(0.00)
Other dairy	-0.05	-0.07	0.00	-0.10	-0.06	-0.01	-0.07	-0.01
	(0.03)	(0.04)	(0.00)	(0.05)	(0.02)	(0.01)	(0.03)	(0.01)
Apples	0.01	0.01	0.00	0.12	0.06	0.01	0.07	0.01
	(0.03)	(0.04)	(0.00)	(0.05)	(0.03)	(0.01)	(0.03)	(0.01)
Bananas	0.01	0.02	0.00	0.19	0.10	0.02	0.12	0.02
	(0.05)	(0.07)	(0.00)	(0.08)	(0.04)	(0.01)	(0.05)	(0.01)
Citrus	0.01	0.02	0.00	0.22	0.11	0.02	0.14	0.02
	(0.05)	(0.08)	(0.00)	(0.09)	(0.05)	(0.01)	(0.06)	(0.01)
Other fresh fruits	0.01	0.01	0.00	0.16	0.08	0.02	0.10	0.02
	(0.04)	(0.06)	(0.00)	(0.07)	(0.03)	(0.01)	(0.04)	(0.01)
Potatoes	0.01	0.01	0.00	0.11	0.06	0.01	0.07	0.01
	(0.03)	(0.04)	(0.00)	(0.05)	(0.03)	(0.01)	(0.03)	(0.01)
Lettuce	0.01	0.01	0.00	0.15	0.08	0.02	0.10	0.02
	(0.04)	(0.05)	(0.00)	(0.07)	(0.03)	(0.01)	(0.04)	(0.01)
Tomatoes	0.01	0.02	0.00	0.22	0.12	0.02	0.14	0.03
	(0.05)	(0.08)	(0.00)	(0.09)	(0.05)	(0.01)	(0.06)	(0.01)
Other fresh vegetables	0.01	0.01	0.00	0.15	0.08	0.02	0.10	0.02
	(0.04)	(0.05)	(0.00)	(0.07)	(0.03)	(0.01)	(0.04)	(0.01)

Appendix Table A.10. (Continued)

	With respect to price of							
Demand for	Condiments, sauces, season.	Miscella-neous FAH	Alcoholic beverages	Limited-service FAFH	Full-service FAFH	Other FAFH	Nonfood	With respect to expenditure
Eggs	0.02	0.05	0.03	0.04	0.05	0.01	-0.29	0.03
	(0.01)	(0.02)	(0.06)	(0.08)	(0.09)	(0.02)	(0.32)	(0.05)
Cheese	-0.06	-0.14	0.07	0.09	0.11	0.02	-0.25	0.13
	(0.03)	(0.06)	(0.10)	(0.13)	(0.16)	(0.03)	(0.40)	(0.06)
Ice cream and	-0.06	-0.13	0.06	0.08	0.10	0.02	-0.25	0.12
froz. dessert	(0.03)	(0.06)	(0.10)	(0.13)	(0.16)	(0.03)	(0.40)	(0.06)
Milk	-0.04	-0.09	0.05	0.06	0.07	0.01	-0.17	0.09
	(0.02)	(0.04)	(0.06)	(0.09)	(0.10)	(0.02)	(0.26)	(0.04)
Other dairy	-0.05	-0.10	0.05	0.07	0.08	0.01	-0.19	0.10
	(0.02)	(0.05)	(0.07)	(0.09)	(0.11)	(0.02)	(0.29)	(0.05)
Apples	0.05	0.12	0.04	0.06	0.07	0.01	0.03	0.03
	(0.02)	(0.05)	(0.08)	(0.10)	(0.13)	(0.02)	(0.32)	(0.04)
Bananas	0.08	0.19	0.07	0.10	0.12	0.02	0.05	0.04
	(0.03)	(0.08)	(0.13)	(0.17)	(0.20)	(0.04)	(0.51)	(0.07)
Citrus	0.09	0.22	0.08	0.11	0.13	0.02	0.06	0.05
	(0.04)	(0.09)	(0.15)	(0.19)	(0.23)	(0.04)	(0.58)	(0.08)
Other fresh fruits	0.07	0.16	0.06	0.08	0.10	0.02	0.04	0.04
	(0.03)	(0.07)	(0.11)	(0.14)	(0.17)	(0.03)	(0.42)	(0.06)
Potatoes	0.05	0.12	0.04	0.06	0.07	0.01	0.03	0.03
	(0.02)	(0.05)	(0.08)	(0.10)	(0.12)	(0.02)	(0.31)	(0.04)
Lettuce	0.07	0.16	0.06	0.08	0.09	0.02	0.04	0.04
	(0.03)	(0.07)	(0.10)	(0.14)	(0.16)	(0.03)	(0.41)	(0.06)
Tomatoes	0.10	0.22	0.08	0.11	0.13	0.02	0.06	0.05
	(0.04)	(0.09)	(0.15)	(0.19)	(0.23)	(0.04)	(0.58)	(0.08)
Other fresh	0.07	0.16	0.06	0.08	0.09	0.02	0.04	0.04
vegetables	(0.03)	(0.06)	(0.10)	(0.14)	(0.16)	(0.03)	(0.41)	(0.06)

	With respect to price of								
Demand for	Flour, prep. mixes	Breakfast cereals	Rice and pasta	Non-white bread	White bread	Biscuits, rolls, muff.	Cakes and cookies	Other bakery products	Beef
Proc. fruits and	-0.02	-0.03	-0.04	-0.02	-0.02	-0.02	-0.05	-0.04	0.06
vegetables	(0.01)	(0.01)	(0.02)	(0.01)	(0.01)	(0.01)	(0.02)	(0.02)	(0.05)
Coffee and tea	-0.01	-0.01	-0.02	-0.01	-0.01	-0.01	-0.02	-0.02	0.06
	(0.02)	(0.03)	(0.04)	(0.02)	(0.02)	(0.02)	(0.05)	(0.04)	(0.04)
Carbonated	-0.02	-0.03	-0.04	-0.02	-0.02	-0.02	-0.05	-0.04	0.12
beverages	(0.03)	(0.05)	(0.07)	(0.03)	(0.04)	(0.03)	(0.09)	(0.07)	(0.07)
Noncarb.	-0.02	-0.03	-0.04	-0.02	-0.02	-0.02	-0.05	-0.04	0.14
beverages	(0.04)	(0.06)	(0.07)	(0.04)	(0.04)	(0.03)	(0.09)	(0.08)	(0.08)
Frozen	-0.01	-0.02	-0.02	-0.01	-0.01	-0.01	-0.03	-0.03	0.09
beverages	(0.03)	(0.04)	(0.05)	(0.03)	(0.03)	(0.02)	(0.07)	(0.06)	(0.07)
Sugar and	0.02	0.03	0.03	0.02	0.02	0.01	0.04	0.04	0.15
sweets	(0.02)	(0.04)	(0.05)	(0.02)	(0.03)	(0.02)	(0.06)	(0.05)	(0.07)
Fats and oils	0.01	0.02	0.02	0.01	0.01	0.01	0.03	0.02	0.09
	(0.01)	(0.02)	(0.03)	(0.01)	(0.02)	(0.01)	(0.04)	(0.03)	(0.04)
Soups	0.01	0.01	0.01	0.01	0.01	0.00	0.01	0.01	0.05
	(0.01)	(0.01)	(0.02)	(0.01)	(0.01)	(0.01)	(0.02)	(0.02)	(0.03)
Frozen foods	0.01	0.02	0.02	0.01	0.01	0.01	0.03	0.02	0.10
	(0.02)	(0.03)	(0.03)	(0.02)	(0.02)	(0.01)	(0.04)	(0.03)	(0.05)
Snacks	0.01	0.02	0.02	0.01	0.01	0.01	0.03	0.02	0.08
	(0.01)	(0.02)	(0.03)	(0.01)	(0.02)	(0.01)	(0.04)	(0.03)	(0.04)
Condiments,	0.01	0.01	0.02	0.01	0.01	0.01	0.02	0.02	0.08
sauces, seas.	(0.01)	(0.02)	(0.03)	(0.01)	(0.01)	(0.01)	(0.03)	(0.03)	(0.04)
Misc. FAH	0.01	0.02	0.03	0.01	0.02	0.01	0.04	0.03	0.12
	(0.02)	(0.03)	(0.04)	(0.02)	(0.02)	(0.02)	(0.05)	(0.04)	(0.06)
Alcoholic	0.00	0.01	0.01	0.00	0.00	0.00	0.01	0.01	0.03
beverage	(0.01)	(0.02)	(0.02)	(0.01)	(0.01)	(0.01)	(0.02)	(0.02)	(0.07)

Appendix Table A.10. (Contineud)

	With respect to price of									
Demand for	Pork	Other red meat	Poultry	Fish	Eggs	Cheese	Ice cream and frozen desserts	Milk	Other dairy	Apples
Proc. fruits and vegetables	0.03	0.01	0.02	0.02	0.00	-0.01	0.00	0.00	0.00	-0.02
	(0.03)	(0.01)	(0.02)	(0.02)	(0.00)	(0.03)	(0.01)	(0.02)	(0.01)	(0.07)
Coffee and tea	0.04	0.01	0.02	0.02	0.01	-0.05	-0.03	-0.04	-0.02	0.00
	(0.02)	(0.01)	(0.01)	(0.01)	(0.00)	(0.03)	(0.02)	(0.02)	(0.01)	(0.01)
Carbonated beverages	0.07	0.03	0.04	0.04	0.01	-0.10	-0.05	-0.08	-0.03	0.00
	(0.04)	(0.02)	(0.03)	(0.03)	(0.01)	(0.06)	(0.03)	(0.04)	(0.02)	(0.01)
Noncarb. beverages	0.08	0.03	0.05	0.05	0.01	-0.11	-0.06	-0.09	-0.04	0.00
	(0.04)	(0.02)	(0.03)	(0.03)	(0.01)	(0.06)	(0.03)	(0.05)	(0.02)	(0.01)
Frozen beverages	0.05	0.02	0.03	0.03	0.01	-0.07	-0.04	-0.05	-0.02	0.00
	(0.04)	(0.01)	(0.02)	(0.02)	(0.01)	(0.05)	(0.03)	(0.04)	(0.02)	(0.01)
Sugar and sweets	0.08	0.03	0.05	0.05	0.01	-0.10	-0.05	-0.08	-0.03	0.03
	(0.04)	(0.02)	(0.03)	(0.03)	(0.01)	(0.04)	(0.02)	(0.03)	(0.02)	(0.01)
Fats and oils	0.05	0.02	0.03	0.03	0.01	-0.06	-0.03	-0.05	-0.02	0.02
	(0.02)	(0.01)	(0.01)	(0.01)	(0.00)	(0.03)	(0.01)	(0.02)	(0.01)	(0.01)
Soups	0.03	0.01	0.02	0.02	0.00	-0.03	-0.02	-0.03	-0.01	0.01
	(0.02)	(0.01)	(0.01)	(0.01)	(0.00)	(0.02)	(0.01)	(0.02)	(0.01)	(0.01)
Frozen foods	0.06	0.02	0.04	0.04	0.01	-0.07	-0.04	-0.05	-0.02	0.02
	(0.03)	(0.01)	(0.02)	(0.02)	(0.00)	(0.03)	(0.02)	(0.02)	(0.01)	(0.01)
Snacks	0.05	0.02	0.03	0.03	0.01	-0.06	-0.03	-0.05	-0.02	0.02
	(0.02)	(0.01)	(0.02)	(0.02)	(0.00)	(0.03)	(0.01)	(0.02)	(0.01)	(0.01)
Condiments, sauces, seas.	0.04	0.02	0.03	0.03	0.01	-0.05	-0.03	-0.04	-0.02	0.01
	(0.02)	(0.01)	(0.01)	(0.01)	(0.00)	(0.02)	(0.01)	(0.02)	(0.01)	(0.01)
Misc. FAH	0.07	0.03	0.04	0.04	0.01	-0.08	-0.05	-0.07	-0.03	0.02
	(0.03)	(0.01)	(0.02)	(0.02)	(0.01)	(0.04)	(0.02)	(0.03)	(0.01)	(0.01)
Alcoholic beverage	0.02	0.01	0.01	0.01	0.00	0.02	0.01	0.01	0.01	0.00
	(0.04)	(0.01)	(0.03)	(0.02)	(0.01)	(0.03)	(0.02)	(0.02)	(0.01)	(0.01)

	With respect to price of								
Demand for	Bananas	Citrus .	Other fresh fruits	Potatoes	Lettuce	Tomatoes	Other fresh vegetable	Processed fruits and vegetables	Coffee and tea
Proc. fruits and vegetables	0.02	0.01	0.20	0.01	0.02	-0.14	0.06	-0.77	0.00
	(0.08)	(0.06)	(0.11)	(0.07)	(0.04)	(0.05)	(0.11)	(0.20)	(0.01)
Coffee and tea	0.00	0.00	0.01	0.00	0.00	0.00	0.01	0.01	-0.12
	(0.01)	(0.01)	(0.02)	(0.01)	(0.01)	(0.01)	(0.02)	(0.02)	(0.21)
Carbonated beverages	0.00	0.01	0.01	0.00	0.00	0.01	0.01	0.01	-0.01
	(0.02)	(0.03)	(0.04)	(0.01)	(0.01)	(0.02)	(0.05)	(0.04)	(0.13)
Noncarb. beverages	0.01	0.01	0.01	0.00	0.00	0.01	0.01	0.01	-0.07
	(0.02)	(0.03)	(0.05)	(0.01)	(0.01)	(0.03)	(0.05)	(0.05)	(0.11)
Frozen beverages	0.00	0.00	0.01	0.00	0.00	0.00	0.01	0.01	-0.08
	(0.02)	(0.02)	(0.03)	(0.01)	(0.01)	(0.02)	(0.04)	(0.03)	(0.49)
Sugar and sweets	0.04	0.05	0.09	0.02	0.02	0.05	0.10	0.09	0.02
	(0.02)	(0.02)	(0.04)	(0.01)	(0.01)	(0.02)	(0.04)	(0.04)	(0.02)
Fats and oils	0.02	0.03	0.05	0.01	0.01	0.03	0.06	0.05	0.01
	(0.01)	(0.01)	(0.02)	(0.01)	(0.01)	(0.01)	(0.02)	(0.02)	(0.01)
Soups	0.01	0.02	0.03	0.01	0.01	0.02	0.03	0.03	0.01
	(0.01)	(0.01)	(0.02)	(0.00)	(0.00)	(0.01)	(0.02)	(0.02)	(0.01)
Frozen foods	0.03	0.04	0.06	0.02	0.02	0.03	0.07	0.06	0.02
	(0.01)	(0.02)	(0.03)	(0.01)	(0.01)	(0.01)	(0.03)	(0.03)	(0.01)
Snacks	0.02	0.03	0.05	0.01	0.01	0.03	0.06	0.05	0.01
	(0.01)	(0.01)	(0.02)	(0.01)	(0.01)	(0.01)	(0.03)	(0.02)	(0.01)
Condiments, sauces, seas.	0.02	0.03	0.05	0.01	0.01	0.03	0.05	0.05	0.01
	(0.01)	(0.01)	(0.02)	(0.01)	(0.01)	(0.01)	(0.02)	(0.02)	(0.01)
Misc. FAH	0.03	0.05	0.08	0.02	0.02	0.04	0.08	0.07	0.02
	(0.01)	(0.02)	(0.03)	(0.01)	(0.01)	(0.02)	(0.03)	(0.03)	(0.02)
Alcoholic beverage	0.01	0.01	0.01	0.00	0.00	0.01	0.01	0.01	0.00
	(0.01)	(0.01)	(0.02)	(0.01)	(0.01)	(0.01)	(0.03)	(0.02)	(0.01)

Appendix Table A.10. (Continued)

	With respect to price of							
Demand for	Carbonated beverages	Non-carbonated beverages	Frozen beverages	Sugar and sweets	Fats and oils	Soups	Frozen meals and snacks	Snacks
Proc. fruits and vegetables	0.01	0.01	0.00	0.12	0.06	0.01	0.07	0.01
	(0.03)	(0.04)	(0.00)	(0.05)	(0.03)	(0.01)	(0.03)	(0.01)
Coffee and tea	-0.02	-0.19	-0.01	0.09	0.05	0.01	0.06	0.01
	(0.27)	(0.27)	(0.06)	(0.08)	(0.04)	(0.01)	(0.05)	(0.01)
Carbonated beverages	-0.30	-0.35	-0.01	0.18	0.09	0.02	0.11	0.02
	(0.38)	(0.39)	(0.07)	(0.15)	(0.08)	(0.02)	(0.09)	(0.02)
Noncarb. beverages	-0.27	-0.44	0.02	0.20	0.11	0.02	0.13	0.02
	(0.30)	(0.37)	(0.07)	(0.16)	(0.09)	(0.02)	(0.10)	(0.02)
Frozen beverages	-0.09	0.32	-0.61	0.12	0.07	0.01	0.08	0.01
	(1.09)	(1.30)	(0.91)	(0.13)	(0.07)	(0.02)	(0.08)	(0.02)
Sugar and sweets	0.09	0.13	0.00	-0.56	-0.01	-0.66	-0.74	0.03
	(0.07)	(0.10)	(0.00)	(0.76)	(0.26)	(0.23)	(0.49)	(0.14)
Fats and oils	0.05	0.08	0.00	-0.02	-0.21	-0.16	-0.23	0.03
	(0.04)	(0.06)	(0.00)	(0.29)	(0.18)	(0.11)	(0.26)	(0.06)
Soups	0.03	0.04	0.00	-2.08	-0.47	0.19	0.96	0.06
	(0.03)	(0.04)	(0.00)	(0.74)	(0.31)	(0.60)	(0.77)	(0.28)
Frozen foods	0.06	0.09	0.00	-0.81	-0.23	0.33	-1.05	-0.22
	(0.05)	(0.07)	(0.00)	(0.53)	(0.25)	(0.27)	(0.72)	(0.15)
Snacks	0.05	0.08	0.00	0.16	0.13	0.09	-1.00	-1.14
	(0.05)	(0.06)	(0.00)	(0.70)	(0.28)	(0.44)	(0.70)	(0.46)
Condiments, sauces, seas.	0.05	0.07	0.00	0.84	0.10	0.12	0.13	0.27
	(0.04)	(0.06)	(0.00)	(0.45)	(0.16)	(0.23)	(0.43)	(0.15)
Misc. FAH	0.08	0.11	0.00	-0.09	-0.23	0.15	0.71	-0.02
	(0.06)	(0.09)	(0.00)	(0.48)	(0.21)	(0.19)	(0.41)	(0.10)
Alcoholic beverage	0.00	0.00	0.00	0.06	0.03	0.01	0.04	0.01
	(0.03)	(0.04)	(0.00)	(0.05)	(0.03)	(0.01)	(0.03)	(0.01)

Demand for	With respect to price of							With respect to expenditure
	Condiments, sauces, season.	Miscella-neous FAH	Alcoholic beverages	Limited-service FAFH	Full-service FAFH	Other FAFH	Nonfood	
Proc. fruits and vegetables	0.05	0.12	0.04	0.06	0.07	0.01	0.03	0.03
	(0.02)	(0.05)	(0.08)	(0.10)	(0.13)	(0.02)	(0.32)	(0.04)
Coffee and tea	0.04	0.09	-0.01	-0.01	-0.01	0.00	0.07	0.01
	(0.03)	(0.08)	(0.07)	(0.10)	(0.12)	(0.02)	(0.24)	(0.03)
Carbonated beverages	0.08	0.18	-0.01	-0.02	-0.02	0.00	0.13	0.02
	(0.06)	(0.15)	(0.14)	(0.19)	(0.23)	(0.04)	(0.45)	(0.06)
Noncarb. beverages	0.09	0.20	-0.01	-0.02	-0.02	0.00	0.15	0.02
	(0.07)	(0.16)	(0.15)	(0.20)	(0.25)	(0.04)	(0.50)	(0.06)
Frozen beverages	0.05	0.12	-0.01	-0.01	-0.01	0.00	0.09	0.01
	(0.06)	(0.13)	(0.11)	(0.15)	(0.18)	(0.03)	(0.35)	(0.05)
Sugar and sweets	0.69	-0.11	0.15	0.20	0.24	0.04	-0.45	0.13
	(0.37)	(0.58)	(0.12)	(0.16)	(0.20)	(0.03)	(0.48)	(0.06)
Fats and oils	0.09	-0.30	0.09	0.12	0.14	0.02	-0.27	0.08
	(0.15)	(0.28)	(0.08)	(0.10)	(0.12)	(0.02)	(0.29)	(0.04)
Soups	0.32	0.57	0.05	0.06	0.08	0.01	-0.15	0.04
	(0.59)	(0.73)	(0.05)	(0.06)	(0.08)	(0.01)	(0.18)	(0.03)
Frozen foods	0.11	0.92	0.10	0.13	0.16	0.03	-0.31	0.09
	(0.38)	(0.54)	(0.09)	(0.12)	(0.14)	(0.02)	(0.32)	(0.05)
Snacks	1.10	-0.13	0.09	0.11	0.14	0.02	-0.26	0.08
	(0.61)	(0.63)	(0.08)	(0.10)	(0.12)	(0.02)	(0.29)	(0.04)
Condiments, sauces, seas.	-1.92	-0.28	0.08	0.11	0.13	0.02	-0.24	0.07
	(0.44)	(0.39)	(0.07)	(0.09)	(0.11)	(0.02)	(0.26)	(0.03)
Misc. FAH	-0.19	-1.48	0.13	0.17	0.20	0.03	-0.38	0.11
	(0.27)	(0.59)	(0.11)	(0.14)	(0.17)	(0.03)	(0.40)	(0.05)
Alcoholic beverage	0.02	0.06	-1.15	-2.17	2.37	-0.13	0.31	0.32
	(0.02)	(0.05)	(0.67)	(0.73)	(0.82)	(0.13)	(0.68)	(0.09)

Appendix Table A.10. (Continued)

	With respect to price of							
Demand for	Flour, prep. mixes	Breakfast cereals	Rice and pasta	Non-white bread	White bread	Biscuits, rolls, muff.	Cakes and cookies	Other bakery products
Limited service	0.00	0.00	0.00	0.00	0.00	0.00	0.01	0.00
	(0.01)	(0.01)	(0.01)	(0.01)	(0.01)	(0.00)	(0.01)	(0.01)
Full service	0.00	0.00	0.00	0.00	0.00	0.00	0.01	0.00
	(0.01)	(0.01)	(0.01)	(0.01)	(0.01)	(0.01)	(0.02)	(0.01)
Other FAFH	0.00	0.00	0.00	0.00	0.00	0.00	0.01	0.00
	(0.01)	(0.01)	(0.01)	(0.01)	(0.01)	(0.01)	(0.02)	(0.01)
Nonfood	0.03	-0.06	0.06	-0.03	0.01	-0.02	0.03	-0.03
	(0.01)	(0.02)	(0.02)	(0.01)	(0.01)	(0.01)	(0.02)	(0.02)

	With respect to price of							
Demand for	Beef	Pork	Other red meat	Poultry	Fish	Eggs	Cheese	Ice cream and frozendesserts
Limited service	0.02	0.01	0.00	0.01	0.01	0.01	0.01	0.01
	(0.04)	(0.02)	(0.01)	(0.01)	(0.01)	(0.02)	(0.01)	(0.01)
Full service	0.02	0.01	0.00	0.01	0.01	0.01	0.01	0.01
	(0.04)	(0.02)	(0.01)	(0.02)	(0.02)	(0.02)	(0.01)	(0.01)
Other FAFH	0.02	0.01	0.00	0.01	0.01	0.01	0.01	0.01
	(0.05)	(0.03)	(0.01)	(0.02)	(0.02)	(0.02)	(0.01)	(0.01)
Nonfood	0.08	0.01	-0.05	-0.05	-0.02	0.06	0.03	-0.08
	(0.02)	(0.01)	(0.01)	(0.01)	(0.02)	(0.03)	(0.02)	(0.03)
						0.01	0.01	0.01

	With respect to price of							
Demand for	Beef	Pork	Other red meat	Poultry	Fish	Eggs	Cheese	Ice cream and frozen desserts
Limited service	0.02	0.01	0.00	0.01	0.01	0.01	0.01	0.01
	(0.04)	(0.02)	(0.01)	(0.01)	(0.01)	(0.02)	(0.01)	(0.01)
Full service	0.02	0.01	0.00	0.01	0.01	0.01	0.01	0.01
	(0.04)	(0.02)	(0.01)	(0.02)	(0.02)	(0.02)	(0.01)	(0.01)
Other FAFH	0.02	0.01	0.00	0.01	0.01	0.01	0.01	0.01
	(0.05)	(0.03)	(0.01)	(0.02)	(0.02)	(0.02)	(0.01)	(0.01)
Nonfood	0.08	0.01	-0.05	-0.05	-0.02	0.06	0.03	-0.08
	(0.02)	(0.01)	(0.01)	(0.01)	(0.02)	(0.03)	(0.02)	(0.03)
						0.01	0.01	0.01

	With respect to price of							
Demand for	Milk	Other dairy	Apples	Bananas	Citrus	Other fresh fruits	Potatoes	Lettuce
Limited service	0.00	0.00	0.00	0.00	0.01	0.00	0.00	0.00
	(0.01)	(0.00)	(0.01)	(0.01)	(0.01)	(0.00)	(0.00)	(0.01)
Full service	0.00	0.00	0.00	0.00	0.01	0.00	0.00	0.00
	(0.01)	(0.00)	(0.01)	(0.01)	(0.01)	(0.00)	(0.00)	(0.01)
Other FAFH	0.00	0.00	0.00	0.01	0.01	0.00	0.00	0.00
	(0.01)	(0.00)	(0.01)	(0.01)	(0.02)	(0.00)	(0.00)	(0.01)
Nonfood	-0.02	-0.02	0.01	0.03	0.00	-0.02	0.00	0.03
	(0.02)	(0.01)	(0.01)	(0.01)	(0.02)	(0.01)	(0.01)	(0.01)
	0.00	0.00	0.00	0.00	0.01	0.00	0.00	0.00

Appendix Table A.10. (Continued)

	With respect to price of							
Demand for	Tomatoes	Other fresh vegetable	Processed fruits and vegetables	Coffee and tea	Carb. beverages	Non-carbonated beverages	Frozen beverages	Sugar andsweets
Limited service	0.01	0.01	0.01	0.00	0.00	0.00	0.00	0.03
	(0.01)	(0.02)	(0.01)	(0.00)	(0.02)	(0.02)	(0.00)	(0.03)
Full service	0.01	0.01	0.01	0.00	0.00	0.00	0.00	0.04
	(0.02)	(0.02)	(0.01)	(0.00)	(0.02)	(0.02)	(0.00)	(0.03)
Other FAFH	0.01	0.01	0.01	0.00	0.00	0.00	0.00	0.04
	(0.02)	(0.02)	(0.02)	(0.00)	(0.02)	(0.03)	(0.00)	(0.03)
Nonfood	0.00	0.06	-0.06	-0.08	0.02	0.05	0.00	0.06
	(0.01)	(0.03)	(0.02)	(0.02)	(0.03)	(0.03)	(0.01)	(0.03)
	0.01	0.01	0.01	0.00	0.00	0.00	0.00	0.03

	With respect to price of						
Demand for	Fats and oils	Soups	Frozen foods	Snacks	Condiments, sauces, seas.	Misc. FAH	Alcoholic beverages
Limited service	0.02	0.00	0.02	0.00	0.01	0.03	-0.90
	(0.01)	(0.00)	(0.02)	(0.00)	(0.01)	(0.03)	(0.31)
Full service	0.02	0.00	0.02	0.00	0.02	0.04	0.91
	(0.02)	(0.00)	(0.02)	(0.00)	(0.01)	(0.03)	(0.31)
Other FAFH	0.02	0.00	0.02	0.00	0.02	0.04	-0.32
	(0.02)	(0.00)	(0.02)	(0.00)	(0.01)	(0.03)	(0.32)
Nonfood	-0.03	-0.03	-0.01	-0.01	-0.04	0.03	0.07
	(0.02)	(0.01)	(0.02)	(0.01)	(0.01)	(0.03)	(0.02)
	0.02	0.00	0.02	0.00	0.01	0.03	-0.90

	With respect to price of				
Demand for	Limited-service FAFH	Full-service FAFH	Other FAFH	Nonfood	With respect to expenditure
Limited service	-0.13	0.42	0.01	0.17	0.18
	(1.08)	(1.15)	(0.07)	(0.37)	(0.05)
Full service	0.38	-1.96	-0.01	0.19	0.20
	(1.06)	(1.10)	(0.07)	(0.42)	(0.06)
Other FAFH	0.08	-0.04	-0.43	0.20	0.21
	(0.37)	(0.42)	(0.18)	(0.44)	(0.07)
Nonfood	-0.08	-0.05	0.00	-1.00	1.21
	(0.03)	(0.03)	(0.01)	(0.07)	(0.01)

Notes: Authors' calculations using first-stage elasticities from table 5, second-stage elasticities from tables A.3.-A.9., and Carpentier and Guyomard's formulas for approximating unconditional elasticities of demand, equations 12 and 13. Standard errors calculated using a residual bootstrap (Green, Hahn, and Rocke 1987).FAFH = Food away from home, including limited-service and full-service restaurants; FAH = Food at home.

APPENDIX: DERIVATIONS OF THE GENERALIZED ORDINARY DIFFERENTIAL DEMAND SYSTEM (GODDS)

The GODDS is a reparameterization of a synthetic model developed by Barten (1993) that exploits the fact that the Rotterdam (*R*), the FDLAIDS (*F*), the NBR (*N*), and the CBS (*C*) models can be rewritten so they all have the same right-hand-side terms:

$$\mathbf{y}_R = \mathbf{w}_n d \ln \mathbf{q}_n = \theta_n \, d \ln \mathbf{Q} + \sum_{j=1}^{N} \pi_{nj} d \ln \mathbf{p}_j, \tag{A.1.0}$$

$$\mathbf{y}_F = d\mathbf{w}_n = \beta_n \, d \ln \mathbf{Q} + \sum_{j=1}^{N} \gamma_{nj} d \ln \mathbf{p}_j, \tag{A.1.1}$$

$$\mathbf{y}_C = \mathbf{w}_n(d \ln \mathbf{q}_n - d \ln \mathbf{Q}) = \beta_n \, d \ln \mathbf{Q} + \sum_{j=1}^{N} \pi_{nj} d \ln \mathbf{p}_j, \tag{A.1.2}$$

$$\mathbf{y}_N = d\mathbf{w}_n + \mathbf{w}_n d \ln \mathbf{Q} = \theta_n \, d \ln \mathbf{Q} + \sum_{j=1}^{N} \gamma_{nj} d \ln \mathbf{p}_j, \tag{A.1.3}$$

where w_n is the budget share for good n, q_n is quantity, p_n is price, and $d \ln Q$ is the Divisia volume index.[1,2]

Barten's general model takes the form:

$$\alpha_R \mathbf{y}_R + \alpha_C \mathbf{y}_C + \alpha_F \mathbf{y}_F + \alpha_N \mathbf{y}_N = \mathbf{X\Omega},$$

where $\mathbf{y}_i$, $i = R, C, N, F$ is a $t \times 1$ vector of transformed basic endogenous variables; $\mathbf{X}$ is a $t \times k$ matrix of exogenous price and expenditure variables; and $\Omega = \mathrm{a}_R\omega_R + \mathrm{a}_C\omega_C + \mathrm{a}_F\omega_F + \mathrm{a}_N\omega_N$ and ω_i, i=R, C, N, F compose a $k \times 1$ vector of coefficients. Without loss of generality, Barten set the sum of the a's to one and solved for α_R. Instead of solving for α_R in (A.1.4), Eales, Durham, and Wessells (1997) solved for α_F such that the term on the left-hand side of the final model is the same as the left-hand side term of the FDAIDS (i.e., $d\mathbf{w}_n$):

$$\alpha_F = 1 - \alpha_R - \alpha_C - \alpha_N. \tag{A.1.5}$$

Substituting a_F from (A.1.5) into (A.1.4) and solving for $\mathbf{y}_F$ yields,

$$y_F = \alpha_C(y_F - y_C) + \alpha_R(y_F - y_R) + \alpha_N(y_F - y_N) + X\Omega. \tag{A.1.6}$$

Unconstrained estimation of the as is not possible since α_F is a linear combination of α_R, α_C, and α_N. However, (A.1.6) can be rewritten using the fact that

$$\mathbf{y}_R - \mathbf{y}_C + \mathbf{y}_F - \mathbf{y}_N = \mathbf{0}, \tag{A.1.7}$$

$$(\mathbf{y}_F - \mathbf{y}_C) + (\mathbf{y}_F - \mathbf{y}_N) - (\mathbf{y}_F - \mathbf{y}_R) = \mathbf{0}. \tag{A.1.8}$$

Solving (A.1.8) for $\mathbf{y}_F - \mathbf{y}_R$ yields

$$(\mathbf{y}_F - \mathbf{y}_C) + (\mathbf{y}_F - \mathbf{y}_N) = (\mathbf{y}_F - \mathbf{y}_R). \tag{A.1.9}$$

and substituting this into (A.1.6) gives

$$\begin{aligned} y_F &= (\alpha_C + \alpha_R)(y_F - y_C) + (\alpha_R + \alpha_N)(y_F - y_N) + X\Omega, \\ &= \varphi_1(y_F - y_C) + \varphi_2(y_F - y_N) + X\Omega. \end{aligned} \tag{A.1.10}$$

The nesting coefficient (φ_1 measures the difference between the price coefficients in the FDLAIDS model and the price coefficients in the CBS and Rotterdam models. The nesting coefficient (φ_2 measures the difference between the marginal budget shares of the FDLAIDS model and marginal budget shares of the NBR and Rotterdam models.

Substituting (A.1.0)-(A.1.3) into (A.1.10) and using

$$d\mathbf{w}_n = \mathbf{w}_n d \ln \mathbf{q}_n + \mathbf{w}_n d \ln \mathbf{p}_n - \mathbf{w}_n d \ln \mathbf{M}, \tag{A.1.11}$$

$$\mathrm{d} \ln \mathbf{M} = \sum_{n=1}^{N} \mathbf{w}_n d \ln \mathbf{p}_n + \sum_{n=1}^{N} \mathbf{w}_n d \ln \mathbf{q}_n, \tag{A.1.12}$$

the GODDS is

$$d\mathbf{w}_n = (c_n + \varphi_1 \mathbf{w}_n) d \ln \mathbf{Q} + \sum_{k=1}^{N} [d_{nk} + \varphi_2 \mathbf{w}_n (\delta_{nk} - \mathbf{w}_k)] d \ln \mathbf{p}_k. \tag{A.1.13}$$

where

$$c_n = \varphi_1 \beta_n + (1 - \varphi_1)\theta_n \text{ and } d_{nk} = \varphi_2 \gamma_{nk} + (1 - \varphi_2)\varpi_n$$

are expenditure and price coefficients to be estimated, respectively, φ_1 and φ_2 are nesting coefficients, δ_{nk} is the Kronecker delta, $\mathbf{w}_n$ is a $t \times 1$ vector of expenditure shares for good n, $\mathbf{p}_k$ is a $t \times 1$ vector of prices of good k, and $\mathbf{Q}$ is a $t \times 1$ vector of Divisia volume indexes.

End Notes

[1] Throughout this study, the different types of FAFH are defined by establishment type. Full-service FAFH are establishments that provide food services to patrons who order and are served while seated (i.e., waiter/ waitress service) and pay after eating. Limited-service FAFH are establishments primarily engaged in providing food services (except snack and nonalcoholic beverage bars) where patrons generally order or select items and pay before eating.

[2] For the compensated law of demand to hold using the LES, all goods must be normal and substitutes for each other. The linear expenditure system (LES) also implies that Engel curves are linear. Last, the own-price elasticity of demand for each food is approximately proportional to its demand elasticity with respect to total expenditure (Deaton and Muellbauer, 1980b, p. 66).

[3] Expenditures on food from catered affairs are inconsistent between 1998 and 2009 in that between 2005 and 2009, no expenditures on food from catered affairs were reported. Hence, we exclude catered food from our analysis.

[4] "Unconditional" in this context means conditional on total expenditure on food, alcoholic beverages, and nonfood.

[5] Gao and Spreen (1994) and Heien and Pompelli (1998) argued that conditional elasticities of demand for meat are appropriate when the aggregate price elasticity of demand for meat is

close to one in magnitude. However, Okrent and Alston (2011) found that the aggregate own-price elasticity of demand for meat is considerably less than one.

[6] Unlike annual data, monthly data could have a unit root at the zero frequency (i.e., standard longrun unit root where first-differencing would have to be applied to render the series stationary) or at seasonal frequencies corresponding to the number of cycles per year. For example, the data-generating process may cycle every 6 months and be nonstationary, which implies that a unit root occurs at that frequency. The goal of the procedure developed by Hylleberg et al. (1990) is to test hypotheses about a particular unit root without taking a stand on whether other seasonal or zero frequency (longrun) unit roots are present. The estimation equations included a constant, a time trend, and lagged dependent variables, and the set of lags was determined using the Bayesian Information Criterion (BIC) and inspection of the partial autocorrelation for each series.

[7] We checked that our estimates were indeed invariant to the equation omitted by arbitrarily leaving out different equations in the first- and second-stage estimation, re-estimating the parameters and standard errors, and recovering the parameters and standard errors of the excluded equation using adding-up. We found our estimates to be invariant to any choice of equation omitted in estimation.

[8] Deaton and Muellbauer (1980a) found that homogeneity is frequently rejected.

[9] Because Edgarton and Shukur (1999) found that the power and size of the Rao-Breusch-Godfrey test deteriorates as the number of equations increases, we also tested for autocorrelation in each equation using the Breusch-Godfrey test and did not find overwhelming evidence of autocorrelation in the first or second stages (see table 4 and appendix tables A.3-A.9).

[10] We estimated ρ to be 0.22 for nonalcoholic beverages.

[11] Bewley, Young, and Colman (1987) developed a measure of goodness-of-fit for a system of equations model as

$$R^2 = 1 - \frac{1}{1 + LR/(T(n-1))}$$

where *LR* is twice the difference between the log likelihood of the model in (1) and the log likelihood of the model with the dependent variable regressed on a constant only. We use a variant of this measure used by Lee, Brown, and Seale (1994) and Brown, Lee, and Seale (1994) where *LR* is twice the difference between the log likelihood of the model in (1) and the log likelihood of the model with the dependent variable regressed on the aggregate income term, d *ln* Q. As Lee, Brown, and Seale (1994) and Brown, Lee, and Seale (1994) showed, this measure is invariant to the equation left out in estimation.

[12] Huang (1993) and Bergtold et al. (2004) are the only recent studies to our knowledge that included a number of disaggregated FAH products in their estimation of unconditional demand systems, such that their results can be compared with ours. Huang (1993) directly estimated demand for 39 foods and a nonfood composite using quantity indexes constructed from per capita disappearance data (ERS) and consumer price indexes. The per capita disappearance data, however, are not direct estimates of retail purchases because they are measured as total commodity supply less quantities used for farm inputs, exports, ending stocks, and industrial uses. Hence, the per capita disappearance data measure food use at a very basic level, do not distinguish between FAFH and FAH, and do not measure use of highly processed foods such as bakery products and frozen dinners in the finished product form (although the ingredients in those products are included as components of less highly

processed foods such as sugar, flour, vegetables for processing, and fresh meat). Bergtold et al. (2004) used price and quantity scanner data (e.g., IRI Infoscan) and the flexible and separable translog multistage demand system (Moschini 2001) to estimate demand for 49 processed foods and an "all-other-goods" composite. One limitation of their dataset is that it did not include information on several key food categories, including fresh meats, fruits and vegetables, and FAFH, and such products were lumped into the "all-other-goods" composite in their model.

[13]The survey reports the mean annualized predictions by professional forecasters of changes in headline (all items) and core (all items excluding food and energy) inflation and personal consumption expenditures (PCE). We used predicted core inflation and headline PCE to proxy for 2012 predicted proportional changes in nonfood price and total expenditures, respectively.

End Notes for Appendix

[1]The Divisia volume index is defined as

$$d \ln Q = d \ln M - \sum_{n=1}^{N} w_n d \ln p_n,$$

where M is total expenditure on all goods. Equivalently, the Divisia volume index is

$$d \ln Q = \sum_{n=1}^{N} w_n d \ln q_n.$$

[2]The coefficient on the income term in the Rotterdam and NBR models (i.e., θ_n) is the marginal budget share and is constant, whereas the marginal budget shares for the FDLAIDS and CBS models (i.e., $\beta_n = \theta_n - w_n$) vary with the expenditure shares. Similarly, the Slutsky terms are considered to be constants in the Rotterdam and CBS models (i.e., $\eth_{nj}$) but vary with expenditure shares in the NBR and FDLAIDS models.

In: Food Away from Home and Food at Home ISBN: 978-1-62808-122-0
Editor: Shane Bauer

Chapter 2

NUTRITIONAL QUALITY OF FOOD PREPARED AT HOME AND AWAY FROM HOME, 1977-2008*

Biing-Hwan Lin and Joanne Guthrie

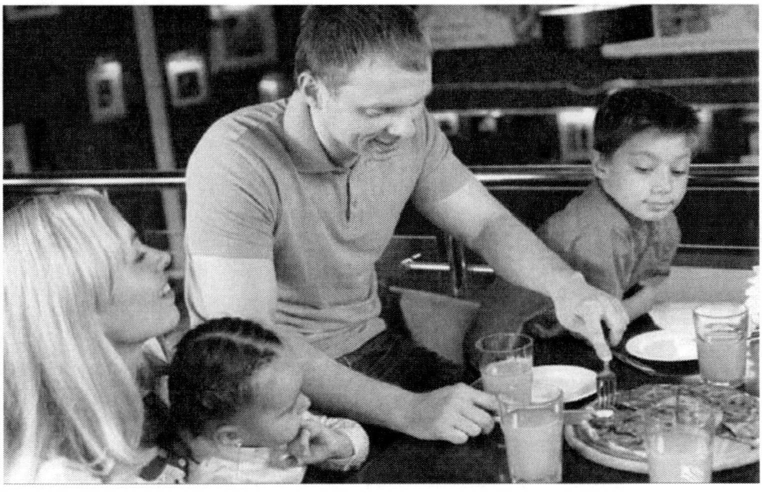

Cover photo credit: Shutterstock.

---

* This is an edited, reformatted and augmented version of United States Department of Agriculture, Economic Research Service, Economic Information Bulletin, Publication No. 105, dated December 2012.

ABSTRACT

Food prepared away from home (FAFH)—whether eaten in restaurants, fast-food and other locations, or as take-out or delivery to be eaten at home—is now a routine part of the diets of most Americans, accounting for 41 percent of food expenditures and 32 percent of caloric intake.

This report analyzes data on individuals 2 years of age and older from two national food consumption surveys (one conducted in 1977-78 and another in 2005-08) to assess changes in the consumption and nutritional quality of FAFH versus food prepared at home (FAH). In the past three decades, FAH has changed more in response to dietary guidance, becoming significantly lower in fat content and richer in calcium, whereas FAFH did not. In 2005-08, FAFH was also higher in saturated fat, sodium, and cholesterol and lower in dietary fiber than FAH. The increased popularity and lower nutritional quality of FAFH is prompting new health promotion strategies, such as menu labeling.

SUMMARY

What Is the Issue?

Food prepared away from home (FAFH)—whether from table-service restaurants, fast-food establishments and other locations, or from a take-out or delivery meal eaten at home—is now a routine part of the diets of most Americans.

Previous Economic Research Service (ERS) research found that FAFH tends to be lower in nutritional quality than food prepared at home (FAH), increases caloric intake, and reduces diet quality among adults and children. This study updates previous research by examining dietary guidance and the nutritional quality of FAH versus FAFH in 2005-08, compared with 1977-78. Poor diets contribute to obesity, heart disease, stroke, cancer, diabetes, osteoarthritis, and other health conditions that impose a substantial economic burden on individuals and society. The increased popularity of FAFH is prompting new health promotion strategies, such as menu labeling, to address this challenge.

What Did the Study Find?

As the share of food expenditures spent on FAFH has risen over the past 30 years, so has the share of calories and nutrients consumed from such food. Previous ERS research found that FAFH in the 1990s contained less of the food components Americans underconsume, such as calcium and dietary fiber, and more of those overconsumed, such as fat, compared with FAH.

Examining the changes in intake from FAFH and FAH, as reported in national Federal surveys for 1977-78 and 2005-08, we found that:

- Americans increased their away-from-home share of caloric intake from 17.7 percent in 1977-78 to 31.6 percent in 2005-08, mainly from table-service and fast-food restaurants.
- Mean daily consumption of total fat declined significantly over the period studied in both absolute terms (grams) and as a share of calories. On average, Americans consumed 85.6 grams of total fat per day in 1977-78, compared with 75.2 grams in 2005-08. The percent of calories from total fat also declined substantially from 39.7 percent to 33.4 percent between 1977 and 2008. Comparing estimates for total fat content between FAFH and FAH shows that the gap has widened over time. Total fat in 1977-78 accounted for 39.6 and 39.9 percent of calories from FAH and FAFH, respectively, compared with 30.5 and 37.2 percent in 2005-08.
- Mean daily calcium intake rose from 743 milligrams (mg) in 1977-78 to 919 mg in 2005-08. For every 1,000 calories from FAH, Americans increased their calcium intake from 425 mg to 559 mg in that time period, whereas the calcium density in FAFH remained relatively constant at 452-460 mg per 1,000 calories.
- Foods obtained at schools had the highest calcium content among all food sources in both periods, but the amount of calcium per 1,000 calories from school foods declined from 742 mg in 1977-78 to 646 mg in 2005-08. The amount of calcium per 1,000 calories in fast-foods increased from 344 mg in 1977-78 to 372 mg in 2005-08.

Data from 2005-08 also included information on saturated fat, cholesterol, sodium, and dietary fiber intake that was unavailable in 1977-78, allowing further analysis of the nutritional differences between FAH and FAFH in the more recent period. We found that in 2005-08:

- FAFH was higher in saturated fat than FAH. The higher percent of calories from saturated fat in fast-foods was especially noteworthy at 13.5 percent, compared with 11.9 percent in restaurant foods, 12.3 percent in school foods, and 10.7 percent in FAH.
- FAFH contained 1,820 mg of sodium per 1,000 calories, considerably higher than FAH at 1,369 mg of sodium. Foods from restaurants and fast-food establishments were particularly sodium-dense at 2,151 mg and 1,864 mg of sodium per 1,000 calories, respectively.
- Similarly, FAFH was more cholesterol-dense than FAH at 144 mg and 126 mg of cholesterol per 1,000 calories, respectively. Within FAFH sources, restaurant foods were most cholesterol-dense at 206 mg per 1,000 calories.
- Even though school foods had the highest calcium content among all food sources, low calcium content in foods consumed at restaurants and fast-food places resulted in lower calcium content overall for FAFH at 460 mg per 1,000 calories, compared with 559 mg for FAH.
- FAFH, especially fast-foods, were lower in dietary fiber (an underconsumed food component) than FAH, 6.8 grams versus 7.7 grams per 1,000 calories.

How Was the Study Conducted?

Our analysis used national food consumption survey data from the 1977-78 Nationwide Food Consumption Survey (NFCS), conducted by the U.S. Department of Agriculture (USDA), as well as data from the 2005-06 and 2007-08 National Health and Nutrition Examination Survey (NHANES), conducted jointly by USDA and the U.S. Department of Health and Human Services, to examine how the nutritional quality of FAH and FAFH has changed. NHANES has been conducted continuously since 1999, however, 2009-10 NHANES data were not released until after this research was completed. Away-from-home sources include restaurants with wait staff, fast-food establishments, schools and day care (for children), and other awayfrom-home places (other). Analyses focused on the nutrient intake emphasized in Federal dietary guidelines for Americans 2 years of age and older. Changes in the consumption of calories, total fat, and calcium from FAH and FAFH sources over the past 30 years were examined statistically. In addition, intake of saturated fat, cholesterol, sodium, and dietary fiber during 2005-08 were analyzed to examine the differences in the nutritional quality of FAH and

FAFH. Our analyses incorporated complex survey design effects and sample weights to estimate population means and test differences in means over time and by food source.

INTRODUCTION

Poor diets contribute to obesity, heart disease, stroke, cancer, diabetes, osteoarthritis, and other health conditions that impose substantial economic burden on Americans (USDA/USDHHS, 2011; USDHHS, 2010). The medical costs associated with overweight and obesity have been estimated as high as $147 billion, or 10 percent of all medical costs in 2008 (Finkelstein et al., 2009; O'Grady and Capretta, 2012; Tsai et al., 2011). These enormous costs are one reason that USDA and other public and private entities place a high priority on improving Americans' diets.

Food prepared away from home (FAFH)—whether eaten in restaurants, fast-food and other locations, or a take-out or delivery meal eaten at home—is now an important part of Americans' diets. The share of total food expenditures spent on FAFH rose steadily from 25.9 percent in 1970 to a peak of 41.9 percent in 2006-07 and then declined to 41.3 percent in 2010 (USDA/ ERS, 2012). Previous ERS research found that, in the 1990s, the nutritional quality of FAFH was inferior to food prepared at home (FAH) (Guthrie et al., 2002). More recent ERS studies found that FAFH increased daily caloric intake and reduced diet quality in both adults and children after controlling for observed and unobserved personal characteristics that could be associated with differences (Todd et al., 2010; Mancino et al., 2010), contributing to poor diet and obesity risk.

Over time, however, differences between FAFH and FAH may change as consumers buy more pre-prepared items in grocery stores, possibly decreasing the differences between the two food sources (Smith, 2010); therefore, re-examination of differences between the two food categories is merited. In this study, we analyzed food consumption survey data collected by the U.S. Department of Agriculture (USDA) during 1977-78 and USDA and the U.S. Department of Health and Human Services (USDHHS) in 2005-08 to examine how the nutritional quality of FAH and FAFH has changed over the past 30 years. Data on three dietary components that have received considerable attention as a part of public health efforts—food energy (calories), total fat, and calcium—are available for both 1977-78 and 2005- 08, allowing trend analysis. Reducing intake of calories and total fat was a major focus of dietary advice during much of the time period between the two surveys, as was the need to increase calcium intake. Trends in average intake, shares of intake by food source, and nutrient density by food source were compared statistically. Information on intake of four additional nutrients targeted as public health concerns—cholesterol, saturated fat, sodium, and dietary fiber—are available from the 2005-08 dataset. Differences in the FAFH and FAH content of these nutrients in 2005-08 are examined statistically. Comparing dietary quality by food preparation source provides insight into how the impact of dietary advice may be moderated by environmental factors, such as increased availability and consumption of FAFH.

Food preparation sources are categorized into two broad categories: FAH and FAFH. FAFH is disaggregated further into four sources—restaurant with waiter service (restaurant), fast-food establishment (fast-food), school cafeteria and school (day care center),[1] and other away-from-home places (other). We analyzed two sets of nationally representative survey data to report mean nutrient intake by food source for adults and children 2 years of age and older. Differences in intake over time and by food source were tested for statistical significance using SUDAAN software (RTI, 2005) to incorporate survey design and sample weights in the analysis.

Data and Methods

The Data: 1977-78 and 2005-08

Between 1935 and 1998, USDA conducted food consumption surveys to assess the nutritional well-being of the U.S. population. Since 2002, USDA has worked with USDHHS to collect and release "What We Eat in America," a component of the National Health and Nutrition Examination Survey (NHANES), which reports food consumption and nutrient intake data from a nationally representative sample of Americans (USDHHS, 2005-06 and 2007-08).

In this study, we analyzed consumption data from USDA's 1977-78 Nationwide Food Consumption Survey (NFCS) as well as from the two most recent cycles of NHANES—2005-06 and 2007-08—available at the time of our analysis.

The 1977-78 NFCS collected food intake data for 3 consecutive days, and the 2005-08 NHANES recorded 2 nonconsecutive days of food intake data. In both surveys, respondents were interviewed in person to collect intake data for the first day, whereas intake information on subsequent days was collected using different methodologies (a self-reported food diary in 1977-78 versus a telephone interview in 2005-08). We analyzed only first-day data to minimize potential bias that may have occurred due to differences in timing (consecutive versus nonconsecutive days) and data collection methods (Cavadini et al., 2000).

Because the Federal *Dietary Guidelines for Americans* (USDHHS/USDA, 2011) do not apply to individuals under 2 years of age, infants and toddlers were excluded from the analysis, resulting in 18,285 respondents from the 2005-08 NHANES and 29,402 respondents from the 1977-78 NFCS.

The surveys collected data on the types and amounts of foods individuals ate and where the food was obtained; using this information, calorie and nutrient intake data were calculated by USDA. The distinction between food at home (FAH) and food away from home (FAFH) in the study was based on where the food was obtained, not where it was eaten. FAH is purchased at retailers, such as a grocery store, a convenience store, or a supermarket; it may be eaten at home or away, as in a brown-bag lunch. FAFH is purchased mainly from foodservice establishments and is further disaggregated into four sources—restaurant, fast-food, school, and other. It may be eaten at one of those establishments or eaten at home, as with a delivery or take-out meal.

Food consumption survey methodology has improved over the past three decades. Some methodological changes may have contributed to the differences reported here:

- A five-step Automated Multiple-Pass Method (AMPM) improves the completeness of data collection and has been employed in NHANES but not in NFCS (Raper et al., 2004). Adopting AMPM may reduce underreporting, resulting in an increase in reported food intake, but the extent of its contribution is unknown.
- Food sources have been expanded, and Hispanic names of eating occasions have been added in NHANES. Because eating occasions are not defined for the respondents, interpretations of eating-occasion names may play a role in the observed differences in meal eating patterns. Consequently, we chose not to report meal eating patterns and nutritional quality by meal occasion in this report.[2]

Methods

Both NFCS and NHANES employed complex survey designs and provided sample weights to generate nationally representative projections. We used SUDAAN statistical software (RTI, 2005) to incorporate survey design effects and sample weights to generate estimates of means and standard errors. NFCS and NHANES were treated as independent samples to test the differences in means for the two periods or by food sources.

There are two approaches to estimating population means and proportions (Freedman et al., 2008). We used the mean approach, in which, for a given nutrient value (e.g., FAFH's share of calories), we calculated the share for each respondent and then calculated the weighted average using sample weights. Alternatively, the weighted sum of a variable (e.g., calories from FAFH) can be calculated and then totaled in a first step, and then the analyst can take the ratio—the ratio approach. These two approaches often yield similar results, although they may produce different but equally valid results (Krebs-Smith et al., 1989).

Observed changes in dietary patterns over time may come from a variety of sources, including an aging U.S. population, the changing racial and ethnic makeup of the U.S. population, and other socioeconomic factors that may influence food consumption decisions. In this study, we compared mean dietary patterns for the two periods without adjusting for changing age, racial, and ethnic composition over time. Further research would be needed to identify the role of such factors.

CHANGES IN THE NUTRITIONAL QUALITY OF FOOD PREPARED AT HOME AND AWAY FROM HOME: 1977-2008

Seven dietary components were examined in the study, including calories, total fat, saturated fat, cholesterol, sodium, dietary fiber, and calcium. In 1980, the Federal Government began publishing the *Dietary Guidelines for Americans*, a set of recommendations to the U.S. population for healthy eating that is updated every 5 years. Over most of the period studied, these guidelines encouraged Americans to control their caloric intake to maintain or achieve healthy weight, moderate total fat, reduce saturated fat, cholesterol, and sodium, and increase calcium and fiber intake (Davis and Saltos, 1999; USDA/USDHHS, 2005). Of these targeted nutrients, only calories, total fat, and calcium were reported in the 1977-78 NFCS. Our discussion focuses first on the intake trends for calories, total fat, and calcium between 1977 and 2008, followed by a discussion of intake during 2005-08 of all the food components examined in this study.

Food Prepared Away from Home Grabs a Larger Share of Caloric Intake

Estimated caloric intake rose significantly from 1,875 calories a day during 1977-78 to 2,002 calories in 2005-08 (table 1). It should be noted, however, that improved survey methodology could contribute to the increase in reported caloric intake. Americans increased their shares of caloric intake from FAFH, from 17.7 percent in 1977-78 to 31.6 percent in 2005-08 (table 2, fig. 1). During 1977-2008, the share of calories from restaurants doubled (from 3.3 to 6.7 percent) and fast-food places registered a four-fold increase (from 3.1 to 13.2 percent). School's share of total caloric intake rose to 3.7 percent in 2005-08 from 3.0 percent in 1977-78.

Table 1. U.S. mean daily caloric and nutrient intakes of individuals 2 years of age and older, 1977-78 and 2005-08

Nutrient	Period	Mean	SE
	1977-78	1,875.12	12.84
Calories (kcal)			
	2005-08	2,002.46	12.29
	1977-78	85.63	0.85
Total fat (grams)			
	2005-08	75.19	0.66
	1977-78	743.45	11.58
Calcium (milligrams)			
	2005-08	918.61	8.47
Saturated fat (grams)	2005-08	25.45	0.23
Cholesterol (milligrams)	2005-08	259.26	2.37
Sodium (milligrams)	2005-08	3,085.15	21.42
Dietary fiber (grams)	2005-08	13.91	0.14

SE = Standard error of the mean. kcal = Kilocalories.

Note: The sample size for 1977-78 was 29,402 and for 2005-08 was 18,285.

Source: First-day intake from the USDA 1977-78 Nationwide Food Consumption Survey and the USDA/USDHHS 2005-08 National Health and Nutrition Examination Survey.

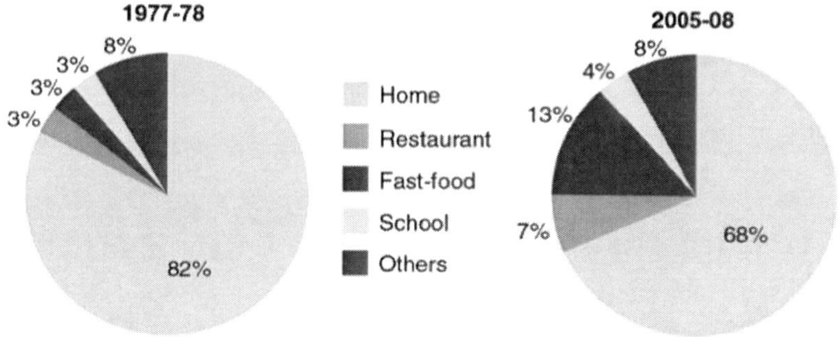

Source: USDA, Economic Research Service analysis using 1977-78 Nationwide Food Consumption Survey data and 2005-08 National Health and Nutrition Examination Survey data.

Figure 1. Between 1977-78 and 2005-08, food away from home (particularly fast-food) increased its share of calories.

Intake of Total Fat Fell Substantially

U.S. daily intake of total fat for individuals 2 years of age and older declined significantly from 85.6 grams in 1977-78 to 75.2 grams in 2005-08 (see table 1). FAFH's share of total fat intake rose proportionally more than the increase in its share of caloric intake during 1977-2008. The largest change was seen in fast-food, which accounted for 3.2 percent of the total fat intake in 1977-78, whereas the share rose to 15.8 percent in 2005-08 (see table 2).

The gap in total fat content between FAH and FAFH was almost nonexistent in 1977-78 but has since widened. In 1977-78, total fat accounted for 39.6 and 39.9 percent of caloric intake from FAH and FAFH foods, respectively (table 3). In 2005-08, total fat accounted for 30.5 and 37.2 percent of total calories from FAH and FAFH, respectively. Food consumed at restaurants had the highest total fat content (44.8 percent of calories from total fat) in 1977-78, but their fat content declined over time and was surpassed by fast-foods in 2005-08. Fast-food places are the only food source from which foods have become more fat dense over time, rising from 40.3 percent of calories from fat in 1977-78 to 41.1 percent in 2005-08. In contrast, the fat content of foods consumed at schools declined over time, from 39.9 percent of calories from total fat in 1977-78 to 33.6 percent in 2005-08.

Table 2. Average shares of U.S. caloric and nutrient intakes, by food source, for individuals 2 years of age and older, 1977-78 and 2005-08

Source	Calories		Total fat		Calcium		Saturated fat		Cholesterol		Sodium		Fiber	
	Mean %	SE	Mean %	SE	Mean %	SE	Mean %	SE	Mean %	SE	Mean %	SE	Mean %	SE
Home														
1977-78	82.28	0.40	81.94	0.40	83.14	0.35	na		na		na		na	
2005-08	68.45	0.44	65.10	0.49	70.26	0.42	65.68	0.48	63.91	0.54	64.14	0.48	68.61	0.45
Away from home:														
1977-78	17.72	0.40	18.06	0.40	16.86	0.35	na		na		na		na	
2005-08	31.55	0.44	34.90	0.49	29.74	0.42	34.32	0.48	36.09	0.54	35.86	0.48	31.39	0.45
Restaurant														
1977-78	3.27	0.22	3.52	0.23	2.86	0.20	na		na		na		na	
2005-08	6.72	0.19	7.47	0.22	5.36	0.16	7.09	0.20	8.76	0.25	8.16	0.25	6.90	0.19
Fast-food														
1977-78	3.11	0.11	3.21	0.12	2.74	0.10	na		na		na		na	
2005-08	13.17	0.27	15.78	0.32	11.66	0.25	15.50	0.32	16.13	0.35	15.59	0.31	13.20	0.28
School														
1977-78	2.95	0.14	3.08	0.14	3.68	0.15	na		na		na		na	
2005-08	3.65	0.21	3.78	0.23	4.45	0.25	3.95	0.23	3.89	0.23	3.88	0.24	3.89	0.24
Others														
1977-78	8.40	0.26	8.24	0.25	7.59	0.24	na		na		na		na	
2005-08	8.00	0.22	7.86	0.23	8.28	0.18	7.78	0.23	7.32	0.25	8.24	0.23	7.39	0.21

na = Not available. SE = Standard error of the mean.

Note: The sample size for 1977-78 was 29,402 and for 2005-08 was 18,285.

Source: First-day intake from the USDA 1977-78 Nationwide Food Consumption Survey and the USDA/USDHHS 2005-08 National Health and Nutrition Examination Survey.

Table 3. Average nutrient density, by food source, for U.S. individuals 2 years of age and older, 1977-78 and 2005-08

	Total fat		Calcium		Saturated fat		Cholesterol		Sodium		Fiber	
Source	Mean	SE	Mean	SE	Mean	SE	Mean	SE	Mean	SE	Mean	SE
	Percent kcal		*mg/1,000 kcal*		*Percent kcal*		*mg/1,000 kcal*		*mg/1,000 kcal*		*g/1,000 kcal*	
Total												
1977-78	39.72	0.17	405.80	3.97	na		na		na		na	
2005-08	33.39	0.14	488.41	3.38	11.37	0.06	130.30	1.23	1,535.80	5.69	7.24	0.06
Home												
1977-78	39.61	0.17	425.38	3.85	na		na		na		na	
2005-08	30.45	0.17	558.91	10.38	10.68	0.07	126.21	1.68	1,368.87	6.86	7.71	0.07
Away from home:												
1977-78	39.93	0.19	451.71	9.20	na		na		na		na	
2005-08	37.23	0.17	459.86	23.29	12.36	0.06	143.97	1.56	1,820.17	12.59	6.78	0.06
Restaurant												
1977-78	44.78	0.37	325.06	4.55	na		na		na		na	
2005-08	38.34	0.40	332.14	6.69	11.85	0.16	205.89	3.98	2,151.42	24.72	7.47	0.11
Fast-food												
1977-78	40.25	0.25	343.60	9.65	na		na		na		na	
2005-08	41.05	0.17	372.43	5.76	13.47	0.07	143.11	1.61	1,864.29	16.65	5.94	0.06
School												
1977-78	39.90	0.22	741.74	20.76	na		na		na		na	
2005-08	33.62	0.35	645.66	16.55	12.28	0.13	111.96	3.42	1,609.49	22.12	7.67	0.20
Others												
1977-78	38.13	0.28	438.05	9.44	na		na		na		na	
2005-08	31.46	0.32	645.11	65.29	11.33	0.14	127.91	3.64	1,591.37	56.63	7.69	0.13

na = Not available. SE = Standard error of the mean. kcal = Kilocalories. mg = Milligrams. g = Grams. Note: The sample size for 1977-78 was 29,402 and for 2005-08 was 18,285.

Source: First-day intake from the USDA 1977-78 Nationwide Food Consumption Survey and the USDA/USDHHS 2005-08 National Health and Nutrition Examination Survey.

During the period studied, school foods may have changed in response to the Healthy Meals for Healthy Americans Act of 1994 (Public Law 103-448), which required the National School Lunch and School Breakfast Programs to meet standards based on the 1990 edition of the *Dietary Guidelines for Americans*, including the requirement that no more than 30 percent of the calories in a meal come from total fat (Ralston et al., 2008).

Calcium Density Fell for School Foods

Mean calcium intake rose significantly from 743 mg a day in 1977-78 to 919 mg in 2005-08 (see table 1). Mirroring the increasing popularity of eating out, the FAFH share of calcium intake rose significantly from 16.9 percent in 1977-78 to 29.7 percent in 2005-08 (see table 2). The calcium density of FAH rose significantly from 425 mg per 1,000 calories in 1977-78 to 559 mg in 2005-08 (see table 3, fig. 2). The calcium density of FAFH, however, has remained essentially constant over time; the increase from 452 mg to 460 mg per 1,000 calories between 1977 and 2008 was not statistically significant.

Examining different sources of FAFH reveals disparate trends. The calcium density of restaurant foods has remained constant; whereas foods consumed at fast-food places have become more calcium dense, rising significantly from 344 mg to 372 mg per 1,000 calories between 1977 and 2008 (see table 3). This increase was offset by a decline in calcium density of foods obtained at school.

Because milk is a required food component in the USDA National School Lunch Program, previous research has shown that foods consumed at school cafeterias have the highest calcium density among all food sources (Lin et al., 1999). The calcium density of school foods dropped significantly, however, from 742 mg to 646 mg per 1,000 calories between 1977 and 2008 (see table 3). This is consistent with declining average milk consumption among children and the proportion of children consuming milk over time (Lin and Ralston, 2003). These changes may be attributable to the increased availability of non-USDA foods and beverages for sale in schools (so called "competitive foods") over this period (Poppendieck, 2010). Substitution of these competitive foods and beverages (e.g., sugar-sweetened beverages in place of milk) may have led to the lower calcium density of foods obtained at school. Schools are the only food source for which calcium density has declined, and the drop is noteworthy at 13 percent.

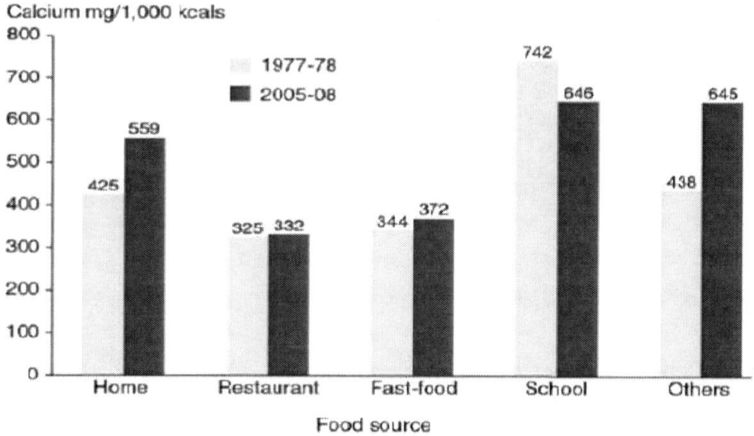

mg=Miligrams.
kcals=Kilocalories.
Source: USDA, Economic Research Service analysis using 1977-78 Nationwide Food.

NUTRITIONAL QUALITY OF FOODS, BY FOOD SOURCE: 2005-08

In addition to calorie, fat, and calcium data, the 2005-08 NHANES included information on intake of saturated fat, cholesterol, sodium, and dietary fiber that was not available in the 1977-78 NFCS. This allowed us to conduct more extensive comparisons of food quality by food preparation source in the more recent period.

Away-from-Home Food Sources Are High in Overconsumed Food Components

During 2005-08, FAFH foods accounted for 31.6 percent of caloric intake and 34.9 percent of total fat intake (see table 2), indicating that FAFH foods are higher in fat than FAH. In fact, the shares of total fat intake from restaurant, fast-food, and school sources were all higher than their shares of caloric intake. There are 11 pair-wise differences in total fat content by various food sources; each pair-wise difference was statistically significant at the 1-percent or better probability level (table 4). Fast-food had the highest total fat content at 41.1 percent, followed by restaurant and school foods at 38.3 and 33.6 percent, respectively, as compared with 30.5 percent for home foods.

Similarly, FAFH foods were higher in saturated fat content than home foods (12.4 versus 10.7 percent of caloric intake), and fast-food had the highest saturated fat content (13.5 percent) among all food sources, followed by schools and restaurants (12.3 and 11.9 percent, respectively). As in the case of total fat, each pair-wise difference in saturated fat content by food source was statistically significant at the 1-percent probability level, except for the differences between restaurants and schools and between restaurants and other FAFH sources, which were significant at the 5-percent level (table 4).

Americans 2 years of age and older consumed an average of 259 mg of cholesterol per day during 2005-08 (see table 1), below the 300-mg-per-day limit recommended by Federal dietary guidance (USDA/USDHHS, 2010). Each of the 11 pair-wise differences in cholesterol density by food source was statistically significant at the 1-percent level, except for home foods and other FAFH foods (table 4). For every 1,000 calories of intake, restaurant foods contained 206 mg of cholesterol, fast-foods contained 143 mg, and other FAFH contained 128 mg. School foods had the lowest cholesterol density (112 mg per 1,000 calories) followed by home foods (126 mg per 1,000 calories).

Individuals 2 years of age and older consumed an average of 3,085 mg of sodium per day during 2005-08 (see table 1), compared with the current Federal dietary recommendation of less than 2,300 mg per day (USDA/USDHHS, 2011). As with total fat, saturated fat, and cholesterol, FAFH foods are more sodium dense than FAH. With the exception of the difference between foods consumed at school and other FAFH sources, each pair-wise difference by food source was statistically significant at the 1-percent level. For each 1,000 calories of intake, foods consumed in restaurants and fast-food places contained 2,151 mg and 1,864 mg of sodium, respectively, compared with 1,369 mg in home foods (see table 3, fig. 3).

Away-from-Home Foods Are Low in Calcium and Dietary Fiber

For every 1,000 calories consumed during 2005-08, FAH contained 559 mg of calcium, which was 22 percent higher than the 460 mg per 1,000 calories in FAFH foods as a whole (see table 3). School foods had the highest calcium density (646 mg per 1,000 calories), compared with fast-food establishments and restaurants (372 mg and 332 mg, respectively).

Table 4. Statistical significance of differences in nutrient density, by food source, 2005-08

			Home			Restaurant			Fast-food		School
Nutrient	All away	Restaurant	Fast-food	School	Other FAFH	Fast-food	School	Other FAFH	School	Other FAFH	Other FAFH
Total fat											
T-statistic	-28.74	-18.11	-44.47	-8.11	-2.80	-6.19	8.82	13.40	18.96	26.50	4.54
Significant level	0.00	0.00	0.00	0.00	0.01	0.00	0.00	0.00	0.00	0.00	0.00
Calcium											
T-statistic	3.88	18.37	15.71	-4.44	-1.30	-4.56	-17.57	-4.77	-15.60	-4.16	0.01
Significant level	0.00	0.00	0.00	0.00	0.19	0.00	0.00	0.00	0.00	0.00	0.99
Saturated fat											
T-statistic	-17.67	-6.67	-27.64	-10.53	-4.18	-9.32	-2.07	2.43	7.89	13.73	4.91
Significant level	0.00	0.00	0.00	0.00	0.00	0.00	0.04	0.02	0.00	0.00	0.00
Cholesterol											
T-statistic	-7.75	-18.46	-7.27	3.75	-0.42	14.63	17.91	14.46	8.25	3.82	-3.19
Significant level	0.00	0.00	0.00	0.00	0.67	0.00	0.00	0.00	0.00	0.00	0.00
Sodium											
T-statistic	-31.47	-30.50	-27.50	-10.39	-3.90	9.63	16.34	9.06	9.20	4.62	0.30
Significant level	0.00	0.00	0.00	0.00	0.00	0.00	0.00	0.00	0.00	0.00	0.77
Dietary fiber											
T-statistic	10.27	1.84	19.03	0.17	0.12	11.96	-0.92	-1.32	-8.48	-12.32	-0.07
Significant level	0.00	0.07	0.00	0.87	0.90	0.00	0.35	0.19	0.00	0.00	0.94

FAFH = Food prepared away from home.

Note: The tests are based on the means, standard errors of the mean, and the sample size (18,285).

Source: First-day intake from the USDA/USDHHS 2005-08 National Health and Nutrition Examination Survey.

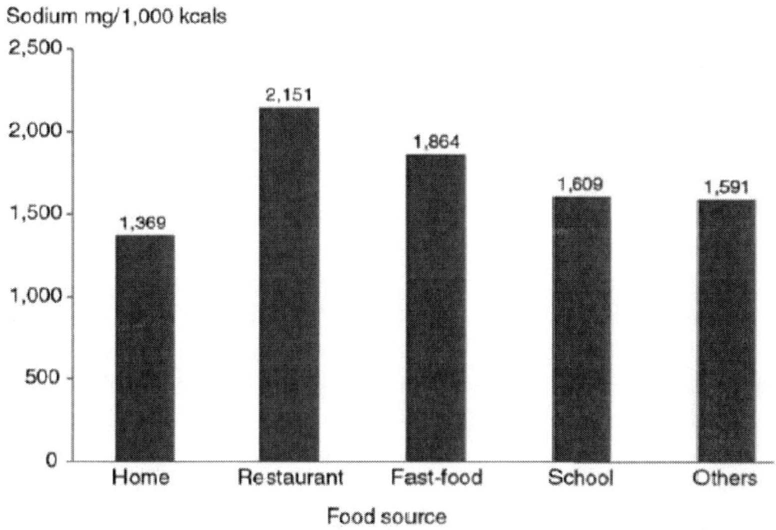

mg=Miligrams.
kcals=Kilocalories.
Source: USDA, Economic Research Service analysis using 2005-08 National Health and Nutrition Examination Survey data.

Figure 3. Restaurants offered the most sodium-dense foods in 2005-08.

FAH was also higher in dietary fiber density than FAFH (7.7 compared with 6.8 grams per 1,000 calories), mainly because of the low fiber density of fast-food (5.9 grams). There was no significant difference in the fiber density of FAH and that of food consumed at schools and other FAFH places. The fiber density of restaurant foods was slightly lower than the fiber density of foods made at home; the difference was significant at the 10-percent level.

DISCUSSION

Over the past 30 years, food prepared away from home (FAFH) has become a regular part of most Americans' diets, and those who monitor food trends expect this to continue (Balzer, 2012). FAFH accounted for 41 percent of food spending in 2008 (USDA/ERS, 2012) and contributed 32 percent of caloric intake, based on our analysis. Unfortunately, consumption of FAFH has been found to increase caloric intake and reduce diet quality in both adults and children (Todd et al., 2010; Mancino et al., 2010).

Poor diets contribute to obesity, heart disease, stroke, cancer, diabetes, osteoarthritis, and other health conditions that impose substantial economic burdens on individuals and society (USDA/USDHHS, 2011; USDHHS, 2010). With estimates of the medical costs associated with overweight and obesity in 2008 ranging as high as $147 billion, or 10 percent of all medical costs (Finkelstein et al., 2009), it is not surprising that USDA, USDHHS, and other public and private entities place a high priority on improving Americans' diets.

National food consumption survey data collected in 1977-78 and 2005-08 were used to compare the nutritional profiles of FAFH and FAFH over the past 30 years. In 2005-08, Americans consumed more calories, less fat, and more calcium compared with 1977-78. In general, FAH was more dense in two underconsumed dietary components—calcium and dietary fiber—and less dense in total fat, saturated fat, cholesterol, and sodium compared with FAFH.

Given the current epidemic of obesity among Americans, the higher caloric intake associated with FAFH has drawn particular policy attention. Anderson and Matsa (2011) have argued that this level of concern is exaggerated, as individuals may compensate for higher caloric intake from FAFH meals by eating fewer calories at a later meal. Levitsky (2005), however, in a review of several experimental tests of energy compensation, concluded that compensation for overconsumption appears to be imprecise and suggested that this may explain changes in body mass index (BMI) associated with long-term exposure to environmental factors that encourage higher caloric intake. Because NHANES collects intake data for 2 nonconsecutive days, the data are not suitable for examining the extent of compensation. More research on the effects of regular, long-term consumption of FAFH on caloric intake, diet quality, and weight status is needed, but our results suggest that its association with higher caloric intake and lower diet quality deserves public health attention.

Both FAH and FAFH changed in many ways between the two periods. Over time, FAH has come to include more pre-prepared items, which might make FAH more nutritionally similar to FAFH (Smith, 2010). Despite this continuing trend, the nutritional quality of FAH changed much more than that of FAFH, perhaps in response to dietary recommendations, such as those to reduce fat and saturate fat intake; it also became more calcium dense. Given these differences, many experts encourage Americans to eat more home-prepared meals as a means of improving diets. Time constraints associated with changes in household structure and women's workforce involvement, however, may discourage cooking (Mancino and Newman, 2007). Innovations that simplify and speed food preparation, such as pre-washed, peeled, and/or chopped vegetables (Lucier et al., 2006) and quick, healthy, simple recipes (USDA/NAL, 2012), have become popular and may help address such barriers.

To improve FAFH nutritional quality, not only must healthy food options be available but consumers must respond by making those choices. There are several reasons why consumers might behave differently when choosing and consuming food prepared away from home compared with home-prepared food (Lin et al., 1999). They might have different attitudes about FAFH, considering it a special treat, compared with FAH. Even if they are concerned about FAFH's nutrient content, they might lack the information to make good choices or have fewer healthy options available.

School food is a special case in that schools are more regulated environments. Changes in USDA school meal regulations that occurred in the 1990s appear to have had an effect on the quality of school food, reducing its total fat content. Fat content declined most in elementary schools, where school food services faced less competition from non-USDA "competitive" foods (Newman et al., 2009). More recent legislation, the Healthy Hunger-Free Kids Act of 2010, requires further improvement in USDA school meals and limits the availability of less-healthful competitive foods and beverages (USDA/FNS, 2010). This has the potential to further improve the nutritional profile of foods obtained at school.

Outside of the school environment, other solutions may be considered. One policy change now underway hinges on improving nutrition information. Since the 1990s, most packaged food sold in retail outlets has been required to carry nutrition labeling. This may have encouraged consumers to make healthier purchases. In contrast, consumers may have less knowledge of the nutritional content of food prepared in restaurants and other outlets. In 2010, the Patient Protection and Affordable Care Act mandated that calorie information be made available on menu boards in chain restaurants with more than 20 outlets nationally to provide consumers with nutritional information that may help them make better choices.

Will menu labeling improve food choices? A limited amount of research has been conducted based on implementation of local menu labeling laws. The findings from these studies were not completely consistent, but generally suggested that menu labeling had a relatively limited impact on consumer behavior (Larson and Story, 2009; Lowenstein, 2011). Information may not be the only factor driving differences in consumer choices when purchasing FAFH. As mentioned previously, consumers may have different attitudes about FAFH; they may still consider it an occasional treat for which less nutritional concern is warranted. This attitude may have fit with the eating patterns of 1977-78 but does not match eating patterns today. Nutrition education efforts and point-of-purchase messages raising awareness of the importance of FAFH as a part of the everyday diet may be helpful and increase consumer response to menu labeling information. Menu labeling may also prompt restaurants to offer more healthy options and to reformulate current offerings. A California study found that restaurants were particularly likely to reformulate items high in calories, fat, or sodium in response to the establishment of a State menu labeling law (Robert Wood Johnson Foundation, 2011). Such supply-oriented effects may increase the effectiveness of menu labeling.

Another potential explanation for differences in FAH and FAFH can be proposed based on behavioral economic theory. Behavioral economics posits that visceral factors, such as hunger and sensory stimuli, may overwhelm self-control, resulting in more impulsive decisions that deliver short-term rewards (Mancino and Kinsey, 2008). For example, when hungry, the sight and smell of a high-calorie treat may be particularly irresistible. FAFH decisions are more likely to be made just prior to eating, and thus fall prey to this problem. Current behavioral economic research explores strategies for avoiding these problems, such as pre-commitment. For example, ordering a healthy meal online and picking it up on the way home may help consumers avoid the temptation to choose a less healthy option when standing in line at a take-out restaurant. Behavioral economics also has demonstrated the power of defaults in guiding choice. In response, public health advocates have urged restaurants and fast-food places to make the healthier options for beverages and side dishes the default choice in children's meals, with positive results among operators who have made the switch (CSPI, 2011). Several other strategies based on behavioral economics may encourage healthful choices (Wansink, 2006) and merit further study.

Implementing menu labeling regulations will provide an opportunity to test the value of nutrition information in helping consumers make better choices when eating out. Consumer education, increased numbers of healthy FAFH offerings, and behavioral economic strategies may also help, reinforcing information approaches. Given the importance of FAFH in overall diet quality, the success of such efforts will have important implications for improving Americans' diets and health.

REFERENCES

Anderson, M., and D. Matsa. "Are Restaurants Really Supersizing America?" *American Economic Journal: Applied Economics* 3(1): pp. 152–88, 2011.

Balzer, H. "Is Cooking a Lost Art?"*EatingWell.com*, 2012, http://www.eatingwell.com/food_news_origins/food_news/is_cooking_a_lost_art_a_conversation_with_harry_balzer_c.

Cavadini C., A. Siega-Riz, and B. Popkin. "U.S. Adolescent Food Intake Trends from 1965 to 1996," *Archives of Disease in Childhood* 87(1): pp. 18-24, 2000.

Center for Science in the Public Interest (CSPI). *Literature Review: Defaults and Choice*, 2011, http://cspinet.org/new/pdf/defaultlitreview.pdf.

Davis, C., and E. Saltos. "Dietary Recommendations and How They Have Changed Over Time," *America's Eating Habit: Changes & Consequences,* AIB-750, chapter 2, E. Frazão (Ed.), U.S. Department of Agriculture, Economic Research Service, 1999, http://www.ers.usda.gov/publications/aib750/.

Finkelstein, E., J. Trogdon, J. Cohen, and W. Dietz. "Annual Medical Spending Attributable To Obesity: Payer-And Service-Specific Estimates," *Health Affairs* 28(5): w822-w831, 2009.

Freedman L., P. Guenther, S. Krebs-Smith, and P. Kott. "A Population's Mean Healthy Eating Index-2005 Scores Are Best Estimated by the Score of the Population Ratio when One 24-Hour Recall is Available," *The Journal of Nutrition* 138(9): pp. 1725-29, 2008.

Guthrie, J., B. Lin, and E. Frazão. "Role of Food Prepared Away From Home in the American Diet, 1977-78 versus 1994-96: Changes and Consequences," *Journal of Nutrition Education and Behavior* 34(3): pp. 140-50, 2002.

Krebs-Smith S.M., P.S. Kott, and P.M. Guenther. "Mean Proportion and Population Proportion: Two Answers to the Same Question?" *Journal of the American Dietetic Association* 89(5): pp. 671–76, 1989.

Larson, N., and M. Story. *Menu Labeling: Does Providing Nutrition Information at the Point of Purchase Affect Consumer Behavior?* Robert Wood Johnson Foundation, Healthy Eating Research, 2009.

Levitsky, D. "The Non-Regulation of Food Intake in Humans: Hope for Reversing the Epidemic of Obesity," *Physiology & Behavior* 86(5): pp. 623-32, 2005.

Lin, B., J. Guthrie, and E. Frazão. *Away-From-Home Foods Increasingly Important to Quality of American Diet*, AIB-749, U.S. Department of

Agriculture, Economic Research Service, 1999, http://www.ers.usda.gov/publications/aib749/.

Lin B., and K. Ralston. *Competitive Foods: Soft Drinks vs. Milk,* FANRR34-7, U.S. Department of Agriculture, Economic Research Service, 2003, http://www.ers.usda.gov/publications/fanrr34/fanrr34-7/.

Lowenstein, G. "Confronting Reality: Pitfalls of Calorie Posting," *American Journal of Clinical Nutrition* 93(4): pp. 679–80, 2011.

Lucier, G., S. Pollack, M. Ali, and A. Perez. *Fruit and Vegetable Backgrounder*, VGS-313-01, U.S. Department of Agriculture, Economic Research Service, 2006, http://www.ers.usda.gov/publications/vgs/apr06/vgs31301/.

Mancino, L., and J. Kinsey. *Is Dietary Knowledge Enough? Hunger, Stress, and Other Roadblocks to Healthy Eating,* ERR-62, U.S. Department of Agriculture, Economic Research Service, 2008, http://www.ers.usda.gov/publications/err62/.

Mancino, L., and C. Newman. *Who Has Time To Cook? How Family Resources Influence Food Preparation,* ERR-40, U.S. Department of Agriculture, Economic Research Service, 2007.

Mancino, L., J. Todd, J. Guthrie, and B. Lin. *How Food Away From Home Affects Children's Diet Quality,* ERR-104, U.S. Department of Agriculture, Economic Research Service, 2010, http://www.ers.usda.gov/publications/err40/.

Newman, C., J. Guthrie, L. Mancino, K. Ralston, and M. Musiker. *Meeting Total Fat Requirements for School Lunches: Influence of School Policies and Characteristics*, ERR-87, U.S. Department of Agriculture, Economic Research Service, 2009, http://www.ers.usda.gov/publications/err87/.

Nielsen, S., and B. Popkin. "Patterns and Trends in Food Portion Sizes, 1977-1998," *The Journal of American Medical Association* 289(4): pp. 450-53, 2003.

O'Grady, M., and J. Capretta. *Assessing the Economics of Obesity and Obesity Interventions, Robert Wood Johnson Foundation*, 2012, http://www.rwjf.org/files/research/74094.5743.assessingobesityinterventions.0312.pdf.

Poppendieck, J. *Free for All: Fixing School Lunch in America,* University of California Press, 2010.

Ralston, K., C. Newman, A. Clauson, J. Guthrie, and J. Buzby. *The National School Lunch Program Background, Trends, and Issues,* ERR-61, U.S. Department of Agriculture, Economic Research Service, 2008, http://www.ers.usda.gov/publications/err61/.

Raper, N., B. Perloff, L. Ingwersen, L. Steinfeldt, and J. Anand. "An Overview of USDA's Dietary Intake Data System," *Journal of Food Composition and Analysis* 17(3-4): pp. 545-55, 2004.

Research Triangle Institute (RTI) International. SUDAAN statistical software, 2005, http://www.rti.org/sudaan/.

Robert Wood Johnson Foundation. *Menu Labeling: What Are Restaurants Doing?* 2011, http://blog.rwjf.org/publichealth/2011/11/03/ menu-labeling-what-are-restaurants-doing/.

Smith, D. "The Ultimate Food Fight," *QSR Magazine*, 2010, http://www.qsrmagazine.com/competition/ultimate-food-fight.

Todd, J., L. Mancino, and B. Lin. *The Impact of Food Away From Home on Adult Diet Quality*, ERR-90, U.S. Department of Agriculture, Economic Research Service, 2010, http://www.ers.usda.gov/publications/err90/.

Tsai, A., D. Williamson, and H. Glick. "Direct Medical Cost of Overweight and Obesity in the USA: A Quantative Systematic Review," *Obesity Review* 12(1):pp. 50-61, 2011.

U.S. Department of Agriculture, Agricultural Research Service (USDA/ ARS). Nationwide Food Consumption Survey, 1977-78, http://www.ars.usda.gov/main/site_main.htm?modecode=12-35-50-00.

U.S. Department of Agriculture, Economic Research Service (USDA/ERS). Food CPI and Expenditure: Food Expenditure Tables, Table 10—Food away from home as a share of food expenditure, 2012, http://www.ers.usda.gov/data-products/food-expenditures.aspx.

U.S. Department of Agriculture, Food and Nutrition Service (USDA/FNS). Healthy Hunger-Free Kids Act of 2010, 2010, http://www.fns.usda.gov/cnd/Governance/Legislation/CNR_2010.htm.

U.S. Department of Agriculture, National Agricultural Library (USDA/ NAL). SNAP-Ed Connection Recipe Finder, 2012, http://recipefinder.nal.usda.gov/.

U.S. Department of Agriculture and U.S. Department of Health and Human Services (USDA/USDHHS). *Dietary Guidelines for Americans, 2005*, 6th Edition, 2005, http://www.cnpp.usda.gov/DGAs2005Guidelines.htm.

U.S. Department of Agriculture and U.S. Department of Health and Human Services (USDA/USDHHS). *Dietary Guidelines for Americans, 2010*, 7th Edition, 2011, http://www.dietaryguidelines.gov.

U.S. Department of Health and Human Services (USDHHS). "Nutrition and Weight Status," *Healthy People 2020: Topics and Objectives,* 2010, *http://www.healthypeople.gov/2020/topicsobjectives2020/overview.aspx?topicid=29.*

U.S. Department of Health and Human Services, Centers for Disease Control and Prevention, National Centers for Health Statistics. National Health and Nutrition Examination Survey (NHANES), 2005-06 and 2007-08, http://www.cdc.gov/nchs/nhanes.htm.

Wansink, B. *Mindless Eating: Why We Eat More Than We Think,* Bantam-Dell: NY, 2006.

End Notes

[1] School (day care center) applies to children only.

[2] In addition to eating-out frequency, caloric intake from FAFH and its share of total calories are influenced by portion size and the difference in caloric content of the same food prepared at home and away from home. Changes in portion sizes over time have been studied by Nielsen and Popkin (2003). There are more than 7,000 food items reported in NHANES, and there are additional data challenges in comparing the nutritional quality of the same food prepared at home and away from home. Further research on the factors affecting caloric intake by food source is needed to explain differences.

INDEX

A

B

C

D

E

F

G

H

I

K

L

M

N

O

P

R

S

T

U

V

W

Y